Gestational Diabetes

Dr Paul Grant MRCP is Consultant Physician in Diabetes and Endocrinology at the Oxford Centre for Diabetes, Endocrinology and Metabolism, and Editor-in-Chief of *The British Journal of Diabetes*.

Overcoming Common Problems Series

Selected titles

A full list of titles is available from Sheldon Press,
36 Causton Street, London SW1P 4ST and on our website at
www.sheldonpress.co.uk

Overcoming Common Problems

Gestational Diabetes

Your survival guide to diabetes in pregnancy

DR PAUL GRANT

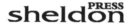
sheldon PRESS

First published in Great Britain in 2016

Sheldon Press
36 Causton Street
London SW1P 4ST
www.sheldonpress.co.uk

The author and publisher have made every effort to ensure that the
external website and email addresses included in this book are correct and
up to date at the time of going to press. The author and publisher are not
responsible for the content, quality or continuing accessibility of the sites.

British Library Cataloguing-in-Publication Data
A catalogue record for this book is available from the British Library

ISBN 978-1-84709-441-4
eBook ISBN 978-1-84709-442-1

Typeset by Fakenham Prepress Solutions, Fakenham, Norfolk NR21 8NN
First printed in Great Britain by Ashford Colour Press
Subsequently digitally reprinted in Great Britain

eBook by Fakenham Prepress Solutions, Fakenham, Norfolk NR21 8NN

Produced on paper from sustainable forests

To Clare, Henry and Molly with love

Contents

Glossary

It's easy to forget that a lot of the time we use medical and technical language that is not familiar or easily understandable. During a degree in medicine it is not uncommon to learn between 20,000 and 30,000 completely new words – this is roughly the equivalent of two new languages. It is unsurprising therefore that when doctors, nurses and midwives communicate with patients there can be confusion and misunderstanding. This is a guide to commonly used medical terms that you may come across in the antenatal diabetes world.

4D scan a new type of ultrasound technology which provides more detail and show's baby's movements

antenatal anything related to the time before birth or during pregnancy or relating to pregnancy

BM the shortcut name given to blood glucose levels (named after the company Boehringer Manheim who used to make the test glucose strips), sometimes also called CBG (see **CBG**)

caesarean section a way of delivering baby – a surgical procedure which involves making a small cut in the lower abdomen in order to get baby out

carbohydrate the name given to sugars and starch within foods which are broken down into glucose in the body and used for fuel, growth and repair

CBG (capillary blood glucose monitoring) the term describing finger prick blood glucose testing from the small blood vessels (capillaries) in the fingertips

CTG (cardio-tocograph) a sensor device usually strapped to your tummy with an elastic belt which allows the midwife to monitor baby's heartbeat during labour and delivery

diabetes mellitus a term generally describing too much sugar (or glucose) in the blood; it does not mean that you are eating too much sugar in your diet, it means that your body is having difficulty controlling the levels of sugar either because there is not enough insulin (see **insulin**) being produced or there is resistance to the action of insulin working effectively

diabetologist a doctor with special training and experience in looking after people with diabetes

fasting a period of time without eating or drinking or relating to the stage just before a meal is taken, e.g. 'the fasting blood glucose level was normal before lunch'

G6PD deficiency glucose-6-phosphate deficiency, a disorder of red blood cells

gestation the period of developing inside the womb between conception and birth

GI (glycaemic index) a ranking of carbohydrate-containing foods, based on their effect on blood glucose levels, from 0 to 100. Pure sugar has a GI rating of 100

glucometer the glucose checking machine, normally a small hand-held device which consists of a digital meter into which test strips are inserted. A droplet of blood is placed on the test strip and the meter then generates a blood glucose measurement value

haemoglobin A1c 'glycosylated haemoglobin' – a measure of long-term glucose exposure

hyperglycaemia a high blood glucose reading. This can affect the unborn baby and can be associated with feeling unwell or irritable, feeling thirsty, increased frequency of urination and blurring of your eyesight

hypoglycaemia a low blood glucose value. This can be associated with feeling unwell, hungry, drowsy and dizzy

induction of labour the action of bringing about labour

insulin an important hormone (chemical messenger) which normally causes glucose from the bloodstream to be taken up into the tissues, such as the muscles or the brain where it can get to work.

Synthetic forms can be used as a medication when an individual is not producing enough of his or her own insulin

insulin resistance is when the body cannot adequately handle high glucose levels due to ineffective action of insulin

macrosomia literally means 'big body' and means a large baby

obstetric relating to pregnancy, childbirth and the processes associated with it

obstetric cholestasis a blockage to the flow of bile from the gall bladder into the gut. There is an increased likelihood of this happening in pregnancy

obstetrician a doctor with special training in how to care for pregnant women and delivering babies

OGTT (oral glucose tolerance test) a special investigation used to see how well your body can handle a set amount of sugar as part of a 'challenge' test

polyhydramnios an excess of the fluid around baby within the uterus which can have multiple causes – gestational diabetes being a common one. The diagnosis is made by ultrasound; the significance can depend on how big the pool of fluid is

post-prandial the time following consumption of a meal. Usually in the context of gestational diabetes, this relates to 1 hour after eating, e.g. 'the post-prandial blood sugars were all high'

pre-eclampsia high blood pressure in pregnancy

premature birth a baby being born more than 3 weeks before it is due; generally this is taken as 37 weeks or less (full term being 40 weeks or 9 months)

Note to the reader

This is not a medical book and is not intended to replace advice from your doctor. Consult your pharmacist or doctor if you believe you have any of the symptoms described, and if you think you might need medical help.

Introduction

Having a baby is one of the most amazing, special and stressful experiences that someone can go through. It can be exhausting, scary and strange, the expectant mother sometimes finding herself veering from glowing with happiness to unexpectedly welling up with tears.

In the midst of this cocktail of physical and emotional stress, a diagnosis of diabetes can come as a bewildering shock and surprise. Gestational diabetes, or GDM, has been around for as long as women have been having babies; however, until recent years, its effects have often been unrecognized and poorly understood and there was no way of testing for it or treating it satisfactorily. It is now thought that GDM affects 15 per cent of all pregnancies worldwide (in India alone there are an estimated 4 million women who have GDM) and there are plenty of famous women out there who have also experienced this including Salma Hayek, Mariah Carey and Angelina Jolie.

Fortunately, we now live in an era where the medical profession and the general public know a lot more about diabetes in pregnancy, midwives are able to screen for it with ease and special antenatal clinics have been set up to allow careful and considerate management of the condition.

If you have recently been diagnosed with gestational diabetes, or are the partner or relative of someone with this condition, the goal of this book is show you that you are not alone. With the right understanding, lifestyle changes and self-management, gestational diabetes can be demystified. The text is framed as a series of (hopefully) straightforward and comprehensive questions and answers relating to many aspects of the condition that come up time and time again. Remember, being diagnosed is a good thing. Even though it will take some extra time and effort to get your sugar levels under control it will be worth it for you and your baby's health.

This book is based on a combination of many years' experience in the diabetes antenatal clinic and the successful multi-disciplinary approach of obstetricians, midwives, diabetes specialist nurses, diabetologists and dieticians working together and sharing the care of women with diabetes. It is with great thanks and respect to the teams in Brighton, Oxford, Tunbridge Wells, and Guy's and St Thomas' Hospitals that this book is jointly dedicated.

There is a glossary at the beginning of the book with explanations for all the words written in **bold type.**

1

Understanding gestational diabetes – what is it and why me?

Elizabeth and her partner, Jon, were very happy to discover that she had become pregnant after months of trying. After the early morning (and afternoon) sickness had settled and the 12-week scan went okay they started telling all their family and friends their good news. They were making plans, cautiously buying equipment for the nursery and debating which pram and pushchair combination to buy.

Claire, the community midwife, was very helpful and explained about all the routine tests and checks that were needed during pregnancy. Elizabeth had initially been rather anxious about labour and delivery as she had some friends who'd had bad experiences, but Claire was able to allay her fears. Elizabeth was fit and healthy and had never been into hospital in her life. Claire talked to her about her personal risks of developing problems during the pregnancy and arranged various blood tests and the like. Elizabeth was sure that there were no major medical problems that ran in her family – but her mum, who had come with her to see the midwife, said that there were a couple of close relatives out there with a history of diabetes and a few big babies had been born recently, including to Elizabeth's half-sister Kate. Because of this background, Claire said that it would be a good idea to screen her for gestational diabetes and arranged to get her tested.

What is gestational diabetes?

During pregnancy (or **gestation**) the human body undergoes many changes and there is a huge amount of metabolic stress due to the significant demands of growing another human being inside you. The normal fuel supply to provide energy and growth is glucose (a type of sugar that comes from **carbohydrates** within our diet), and this is well regulated within a tightly controlled range. The hormone which normally helps to control blood glucose levels is called **insulin** and this is a type of chemical messenger which

1

signals glucose to be taken up into the body's cells and tissues and put to work. More on this subject later.

Diabetes is the name given to the condition which occurs when the body is unable to handle the levels of glucose within the bloodstream and the levels can begin to stray too high above the normal range. When this occurs, most commonly around 28 weeks of pregnancy, it can have implications for the growing baby, the mother and the pregnancy.

Does it mean that I have been eating too much sugar?

No. Glucose is an important fuel that powers the body and comes from carbohydrates in our food (such as rice, pasta, bread and potatoes). It does not necessarily mean that you are eating too much sugar in your diet, it just means that the body is unable to control blood sugar levels within the normal range and this is the essence of gestational diabetes (GDM). It may well be that the insulin which your body is making already is not enough to meet your requirements or that the effects of pregnancy and other important hormones being released are causing your body to become resistant to its effects. The most important thing to realize is that you are not to blame for developing gestational diabetes and with the right support and motivation the challenges of GDM can be met.

Why might I have been tested for gestational diabetes?

Modern pregnancy care is based around reducing the risks for mother and baby. It has been recognized over recent years that there are several factors which increase the risk of developing diabetes during pregnancy, so midwives are trained to recognize both the early signs of diabetes and the potential risk factors which may make diabetes more likely to occur. It is on this basis that individuals are put forward for testing. In the UK there is generally clear guidance over which women should be tested for GDM. These include:

- women with a strong background family history of diabetes (especially in close relatives);

- women who have had diabetes in previous pregnancies, or who have had very large babies;
- women in certain ethnic groups e.g. Afro-Caribbean, south-east Asian, Middle Eastern;
- women who are overweight, generally those with a body mass index (BMI) over 30.

You may be screened for gestational diabetes at your first antenatal appointment with your midwife or GP (the booking visit), which takes place around weeks 8–12 of your pregnancy. At this time, your GP or midwife will find out if you are at increased risk of gestational diabetes. They will ask about any known risk factors, such as whether you have a family history of diabetes. If any of these apply to you, you'll be offered a blood test to check your glucose levels.

How is gestational diabetes diagnosed?

The gold standard for diagnosing GDM is a specific test called an **oral glucose tolerance test (OGTT)**. The test should ideally be done at 24–28 weeks pregnancy, with testing being performed earlier on in pregnancy if the person has had GDM previously.

This is a type of 'challenge test' which assesses how well your body responds to the stimulation of a specific amount of glucose – in this case, exactly 75 grams of glucose in a liquid drink. A blood test is done at the beginning of the test to see what the background blood glucose level is doing (when you have fasted; that is, not had anything to eat), the sugary drink is then taken and then the individual has to sit still or be relatively relaxed for the next 2 hours (to avoid distorting the test results). At the end of 2 hours, a final blood test is taken and the two blood glucose values are compared to see how well the body was able to handle the large glucose load.

The normal range for glucose levels in the bloodstream are roughly 3.0 to 5.0 millimoles (mmol) per litre when a person has not been eating and roughly 5.0 to 7.0 mmol per litre after having a meal. It is natural for there to be a bit of a rise, everyone is slightly different. The cut-off value for diagnosing GDM following an OGTT has traditionally been agreed at 7.8 mmol per litre. If the test has been done correctly with no interference then a value below

7.8 mmol per litre at 2 hours suggests normal handling of glucose (not diabetic). A value greater than 7.8 mmol per litre is diagnostic of GDM. This may seem like a rather arbitrary cut-off but the reason for this value being so crucial is that at this level of glucose intolerance (or glucose mishandling in the body) there is a significant rise in the risk of complications occurring during pregnancy.

Tests which should *not* be used to diagnose GDM include: urinary glucose monitoring, **fasting** blood glucose and random measurements of blood glucose. Some areas do however use the 'Lucozade test' which is an easy-to-perform screening test.

The Lucozade test

This is a screening test which tells us whether you are at risk of GDM. It may be done in your GP surgery or with the community midwife.

- You'll be asked to drink a small bottle of original Lucozade.
- You need to measure out 275 millilitres and drink all of it pretty much straightaway.
- One hour after having the drink you will have a blood test to measure your blood glucose levels.
- During the hour you shouldn't have anything else to eat or drink except for sips of water.

If the results of the test are normal then it suggests that you are at a very low risk of developing GDM and you don't need to do anything else. If the test results are high, then you are at a higher risk for having diabetes and it will be recommended that you go on to have a formal OGTT diagnostic test.

What if I don't want to have the tests?

If you would prefer not to be tested for gestational diabetes you don't have to. However this would be the standard thing to do if you fulfil one or more of the risk categories and there is no other reliable way of telling whether you have gestational diabetes or not. It would be a shame to miss out on the best available treatment if you had diabetes but didn't know, especially when there are such good treatments available and those who are untreated can run into serious problems.

Can there be a mistake with the diagnosis?

The OGTT is a good test (and often considered to be the 'gold standard') but as with anything it is not entirely perfect. Overall, it provides a good picture of your glucose dynamics which is a clever way of looking at how the body is able to control or regulate the levels of glucose in the bloodstream.

Remember, being diagnosed with GDM does not mean that you are a bad person or have a terrible diet or that you have done

Problems with the oral glucose tolerance test

For the OGTT to give us a reliable result it is important that the individual is in good health and that there are no interfering factors (even a common cold can distort the results).

Interfering factors include:

- duration of fasting before the test;
- the time of day the test is performed;
- carbohydrate intake or activity during the test (sitting quietly for 2 hours during the test is recommended).

The test subject should avoid taking any medications which could interfere with the levels of blood glucose and avoid smoking, drinking caffeine or having anything to eat too close to the start of the test. People should fast for at least 8 hours before the test (ideally 12 hours).

It is important to make sure that the right amount and formulation of glucose is given (and all of it is drunk down) – 75 grams of powdered glucose in a set volume of fluid.

The diagnosis of diabetes should be based on laboratory blood glucose values rather than finger prick glucose tests as the former are more accurate.

Failure to realize that the OGTT is being undertaken on a pregnant person can sometimes lead to confusion as the cut-off level for a diagnosis of gestational diabetes is much lower than in the non-pregnant population.

The test results themselves will not indicate whether the organization and performance of the test were carried out correctly. Small errors as suggested above may contribute to an erroneous result.

something wrong, it is just a reflection of the fact that pregnancy is hard work on the body and sometimes the body's metabolism can be put under strain.

Some problems with the test can relate to how the test was performed or some individual factors. For example, making sure that the person is properly fasted before the test (i.e. the person has eaten no food for 12 hours beforehand) is important, as is ensuring that the individual is relatively still and relaxed during the 2-hour test period – not wandering around, or working, or eating snacks, or breastfeeding or chasing after another child.

What do the results of the OGTT mean?

Confusingly, there are two competing criteria which are being used to diagnose GDM following the oral glucose tolerance test, and whether you are diagnosed with GDM will depend slightly on which criteria your local centre uses (Table 1.1). It is always best to speak with your midwife if there is any uncertainty. Some people demand to have the OGTT repeated if there is any controversy. Even diabetes doctors can sometimes disagree over the actual diagnosis!

Table 1.1 Diagnostic levels for the diagnosis of gestational diabetes

	World Health Organization	International Association of Diabetes and Pregnancy Study Group
Fasting glucose level	> 7.0 mmol/l	> 5.1 mmol/l
Post carbohydrate load level	> 7.8 mmol/l at 2 hours	> 10.1 mmol/l at 1 hour or > 8.5 mmol/l at 2 hours

Can I have the OGTT again if I don't agree with it?

Yes, this would be reasonable if there is a problem. Repeating the OGTT because results are potentially incorrect may be considered in at least two circumstances:

- mildly abnormal results and the possibility of incorrect preparation for and/or administration of the test (e.g. as suggested from the patient's memory of the test);

- slightly abnormal results and major implications of abnormality for the person's future life (e.g. loss of job; difficulties obtaining insurance).

Results of the OGTT can change even within the same individual if he or she has it on more than one occasion. There is potentially a variation of approximately 8 per cent for fasting values and of approximately 20 per cent for 2-hour values. This means that in 20 per cent of repeat tests compared to the original values, fasting values will be at least 13 per cent higher or 13 per cent lower and 2-hour values will be at least 33 per cent higher or 33 per cent lower. The sensitivity of the test to incorrect preparation or administration and the high individual variability, unfortunately, make the gold standard for diabetes diagnosis less than perfectly reliable. The sensible thing to do under the circumstances is to discuss the results with your midwife or the consultant diabetologist (they are well used to discussing the vagaries of the diagnosis of diabetes). They may well take a holistic view and suggest that while the OGTT results are equivocal it would be a potentially safe approach to get you to do some daily blood glucose monitoring and then arrange to review the results with you to see if there is a tendency for you to have higher glucose levels.

What about this HbA1c blood test that I've heard of?

It has been recommended by NICE (the National Institute for Health and Care Excellence) that a specific blood test for something called **haemoglobin A1c** (HbA1c) is performed in all women with GDM at the time of diagnosis. This is to pick up those people who may already have type 2 diabetes (but did not realize as they had no obvious symptoms). HbA1c relates to something called 'glycosylation of the red blood cells' (haemoglobin) as a measure of how much glucose there has been around over the last few months within the bloodstream. Red blood cells live for around 120 days on average, whizzing around the circulation picking up glucose as they go. So looking at how 'sugar-coated' they are, acts as a reflection of chronic glucose exposure. One way of thinking about it is by considering the difference between looking at a cornflake and a frostie!

If your HbA1c is below 6.0 per cent (42 mmol/mol) – a newer standardized measurement of HbA1c – then it is unlikely that you have pre-existing type 2 diabetes. If it is in the range of 6.0–6.5 per cent (42–48 mmol/mol in new units) or higher then it is likely that you already have type 2 diabetes. This test does run the risk of missing some people however, as HbA1c tends to fall slightly during normal pregnancy anyway.

Why me?

It may not seem at all fair to be diagnosed with GDM, especially if you are otherwise healthy and this is your first pregnancy. Such a diagnosis can often be quite a shock and cause distress and guilt. It may be that you have one of the many risk factors or come from a family with a strong background of diabetes; sometimes however, no clear explanation is found and this can be frustrating. You are not alone. High glucose levels occur in anywhere from 3 to 5 per cent of women during pregnancy.

On a metabolic level, pregnancy induces an environment of resistance to the effective action of insulin and this is made worse by the increased production of progesterone and growth hormone, placental hormones such as lactogen, and rises in the stress hormone cortisol which also disrupts blood glucose levels.

What are the risk factors for gestational diabetes?

There is a genetic component to diabetes and so those individuals with close relatives (parents, siblings, aunts, uncles, grandparents) who have diabetes are recognized to be at risk. Other well-known risk factors include:

- ethnicity – people from certain ethnic backgrounds have a higher than average rate of type 2 diabetes, e.g. South Asian families, people from the Middle East and Afro-Caribbean individuals;
- being overweight, which is generally deemed to be a BMI above 30;
- having had GDM in a previous pregnancy;
- having had a large baby in a previous pregnancy – 4.5 kilos (8.8 pounds) or more;

- a history of unexplained stillbirth or the baby dying soon after birth;
- there being a higher than average volume of fluid around baby, known as **polyhydramnios.**

How do I know everything is being done in the best possible way?

One of the things that you will pick up from reading this book is that antenatal services differ throughout the country and depending on where you are seen some of the content may be more or less relevant. Different clinicians may treat you in slightly different ways and you may get a different schedule of visits or get more or less intensive care depending on the local set-up. You may have a friend or relative who describes a completely different system of care elsewhere from the one which you are receiving.

Pregnancy is a very important time and fortunately the well-respected organization NICE have spent a great deal of time looking at the evidence base for the various interventions and treatments for somebody with diabetes in pregnancy. The latest set of guidance was updated in early 2015 ('Diabetes in pregnancy: management of diabetes and its complications from preconception to the postnatal period') and can be found at <https://www.nice.org.uk/guidance/ng3> (this makes interesting reading – if you are having difficulty sleeping).

If you are unhappy with any aspect of your treatment at any point – then you must say something. Remember, everything should be in place to support you and if we are getting it wrong on a local level then we need to know. Often your midwife is a receptive point of contact. People are reluctant to challenge their doctors, but comments and suggestions and constructive criticism are the only way we can get proper feedback.

What does the NICE guidance say?

This newest version makes several recommendations, in particular around GDM diagnosis and treatment – NICE agree that the diagnosis of GDM has been plagued by inconsistencies, with the International

Association of Diabetes & Pregnancy Study Group (IADPSG) not recommending universal screening, but rather going for the use of OGTT at 24–28 weeks pregnancy in women with one or more risk factors. The latest advice however for those who have had GDM in an earlier pregnancy is to either have an OGTT or start self-monitoring of blood sugars as early in pregnancy as possible – this approach is useful for helping to identify women who have developed unrecognized type 2 diabetes in between pregnancies and enable them to be started on the right treatment promptly. Each different centre has the option to advise whether they think that self-monitoring of glucose levels should be episodic (i.e. for a week at a time and then reviewed) or continuously throughout pregnancy. Periodic checking would be cheaper for the health service and perhaps less stressful for the individual, whereas constant self-monitoring allows earlier pick-up and intervention for GDM if it occurs.

In terms of the diagnostic levels on the OGTT, the NICE guidance isn't the same as that given by the IADPSG or the World Health Organization (WHO). Instead NICE opts for:

- a fasting blood glucose level at the start of the test of 5.6 or above; or
- an OGTT 2-hour value of 7.8.

The latest version of the NICE guidance tightens up its suggestions for the early management of GDM – stating that the standard should be for the newly diagnosed person to be seen at a joint antenatal diabetes service within one week of diagnosis, that there should be efficient communication with your GP and that dietary input should be triggered straightaway – with a focus on a low **glycaemic index** (GI) diet (lots more on this later). They also now recommend that 30 minutes of exercise after meals should take place. More on exercise in Chapter 5 – this is a good suggestion, but many will find this difficult to put into practice.

What are the NICE targets for treatment?

Again, there has traditionally been disparity over the specific blood glucose targets that we should aim for. The reason for having a target per se is that there will be a greater burden of disease and a significantly increased risk of complications if blood glucose levels are consistently too high. 'Too high' is defined by NICE as being a blood glucose level of 5.3 mmol per litre (mmol/l) or greater before a meal (referred to as being in the fasted state) and 7.8 mmol/l or more 1 hour after eating a meal.

The overall treatment pathway therefore can be simplified to:

1 self-monitoring of blood glucose begins and if the blood sugars are persistently out of target then the dietary and lifestyle changes are implemented and the levels reviewed;
2 if after a reasonable duration, perhaps one week, the glucose levels are too high too frequently, then a recommendation is made for starting on tablet medication (commonly metformin, or glibenclamide for those who cannot take metformin due to any side effects);
3 blood sugars are then monitored and if still not controlled despite stepping up the dose of the tablets then a discussion is had around commencing insulin therapy (as insulin is what the body is lacking at this stage);
4 insulin is then introduced and its dose can be adjusted (or titrated) according to the results of the sugar monitoring (and other external factors such as baby's growth).

One new suggestion in the NICE guidance is that of starting insulin immediately at diagnosis if the pregnant woman's fasting blood glucose level is 7.0 mmol/l or more, as well as in those who are found to have an elevated blood glucose level in the range 6.0–6.9 mmol/l if the growth scans demonstrate that baby is on the large side (**macrosomia**) or there is too much fluid around baby within the womb (polyhydramnios). In some places this occurs already, in others there may be reluctance to institute injectable therapy so soon.

NICE also make recommendations about the timing of delivery and not letting the pregnancy go on too long in order to reduce risks and complications. Those with GDM are advised to give birth no later than 40 weeks and 6 days (an average 9 month pregnancy is roughly 40 weeks) and if a woman has not yet given birth naturally by this stage she should be offered an **induction of labour** (or have a caesarean if required). If there are any complications affecting mother or baby prior to this time, or she is on metformin or insulin, then earlier delivery should be discussed, e.g. around 37 to 38 weeks (more on this in Chapters 7 and 8).

What are the other types of diabetes?

There are several different conditions which come under the umbrella of diabetes. Diabetes is a general term used to describe too much sugar in the bloodstream. The actual word diabetes means 'siphon', so called as the classic description of the condition is of people passing large amounts of urine, like a siphon (liquid passing through a tube). Gestational diabetes describes this process happening solely in the context of pregnancy. Once pregnancy is over, the diabetes goes away – it's really quite remarkable. The other types of diabetes are:

- *Type 1 diabetes* is usually first diagnosed in childhood or adolescence and is caused by failure of the pancreas gland to make enough insulin. Without insulin, blood sugar levels go up and people become unwell. The treatment is to replace the insulin – for life. Currently there is no cure. Young women who already have diabetes are usually counselled about getting ready for pregnancy well in advance by their diabetes specialist nursing team.
- *Type 2 diabetes* tends to happen in older adults and has several causes. Risk factors include genetic susceptibility or family history, being overweight and certain ethnic groups. The defining feature here is insulin resistance. The pancreas continues to work – but not enough to be able to regulate the levels of glucose in the blood. Dieting, tablets and insulin are all used to help control type 2 diabetes. One recognized cure for type 2 diabetes is significant, sustained weight loss.
- *Secondary diabetes* can occur as a consequence of other types of damage to the pancreas; these might include pancreatitis (an inflammation of the gland), cystic fibrosis, or trauma to, or surgical removal of, the pancreas.

Who can I talk to?

Understandably, you may be finding things difficult. It's all right to be uncertain about the changes you'll need to make. It can be helpful to talk things through. It's often good to share your thoughts with family and friends. Your midwife and GP are always good points of call, you will also meet and be given the contact details of the antenatal diabetes team and should be able to speak with the specialist diabetes midwife and diabetes specialist nurse when needed. It's important to remember that you are not alone in this and can call the Diabetes UK Careline on 0345 123 2399 or chat with others on the Diabetes UK forum online. Other good sources of information and support include <www.mumsnet.com> and the InDependent Diabetes Trust <www.iddt.org>.

2

What next? Coming to terms with the diagnosis

Claire, the community midwife, phoned Elizabeth the day after her glucose tolerance test and explained to her that it showed that she had gestational diabetes. Elizabeth wasn't expecting this at all and didn't believe it. She said that there must be some mistake and that either her results had been mixed up with someone else's or that they were only just borderline as she had been stressed during the test. Claire had to calm her and explain that the test result was diagnostic and unfortunately clearly indicated that at that stage of pregnancy she was in the diabetic range.

Elizabeth felt very guilty about this as she now thought that she had personally done something wrong and that her pregnancy had been spoilt by this new condition which she didn't want or feel that she deserved. She was very reluctant to tell her partner but Jon could see that something had upset her.

How common is gestational diabetes?

Gestational diabetes is a common condition, and up to 18 in every 100 women giving birth in England and Wales may be affected.

Can I just do nothing and ignore this?

The key thing to be aware of when told that you have gestational diabetes is that you have the right information. The vast majority of women with GDM have a safe and normal pregnancy and everything goes well with the delivery. However it can be very difficult to predict who is likely to have the mild, moderate or more severe forms of the condition and there is no clear way of predicting the eventual outcome at the time of diagnosis.

Being diagnosed with any medical condition in pregnancy can be difficult to come to terms with and there is often a perception that this wonderful and natural experience is at risk of being medicalized or somehow interfered with. You are well within your rights to reject any input that you are unhappy with and this is eminently understandable.

If you are diagnosed with GDM, your midwife should inform your GP and you will be referred to a specialist joint antenatal diabetes outpatient clinic within one week.

Being informed and asking the right questions are perhaps the most appropriate ways of dealing with the conflicting sensations under the circumstances. Disengaging with the **obstetric** or midwifery team is potentially unhelpful as you could miss out on a wealth of experience and support. Ultimately, being diagnosed is a good thing.

The do-nothing scenario is understandable, but is potentially risky and not advisable. One of the purposes of this book is to try and answer some of the questions that present themselves at this difficult time. Ultimately, if GDM is ignored or not monitored properly then the risks of poor outcomes and complications are significantly increased.

Does this mean I have diabetes for ever?

Good question. For the majority of women, GDM tends to fade away as soon as baby is born. However it may be that the GDM was in fact undiagnosed type 1 or type 2 diabetes picked up for the first time, so people are always checked after delivery to make sure their blood sugars have gone back to normal.

If you consider pregnancy to be the ultimate physical stress test, it demonstrates that when put under pressure the body's handling of glucose goes out of kilter. High blood glucose levels in pregnancy are associated with a higher risk of developing type 2 diabetes in up to 50 per cent of women over the following 10 years. However it is well recognized that the chances of getting diabetes later on are reduced significantly by being able to lose weight, paying attention to diet and lifestyle factors and the use of the medication called metformin (more on this useful tablet later).

What effect will gestational diabetes have on me?

GDM is known to have both physical and psychological effects on mum. It can precipitate a great deal of stress, anxiety and guilt. High blood pressure is a possibility and will be regularly checked for and monitored, and treated if necessary. There is also an increased risk of a condition known as **pre-eclampsia**. Because of some of the risks occurring during pregnancy regarding baby there is also a higher number of **caesarean section** deliveries when compared with non-diabetes related pregnancies.

What symptoms might I experience?

Gestational diabetes often doesn't cause any symptoms. The best way to identify it is with blood tests. This means you may be screened for the condition at your first antenatal appointment by a blood glucose sample from the vein (not a finger prick), at around weeks 8–12 of pregnancy.

If you are at an increased risk of gestational diabetes you will be offered a full test, which takes place during weeks 24–28 of pregnancy.

High blood glucose (**hyperglycaemia**) can cause some symptoms, including:

- a dry mouth with increased thirst
- needing to urinate frequently, especially at night
- tiredness
- recurrent infections, such as thrush
- blurred eyesight
- feeling tired, irritable and rough.

What effects will gestational diabetes have on my baby?

There is a clear relationship between high blood glucose levels and worse outcomes for baby. The excess of glucose in the system predisposes baby to grow more and get too large for the space baby is squashed into. This is known as **macrosomia**, which literally means 'big body'. The delivery of larger babies can then cause problems as the baby enters the birth canal, with damage to shoulders and nerves a possibility as well as the risk of fractures if baby gets stuck.

Overall, there is an increased risk of miscarriage and stillbirth when compared with the non-diabetic population, and a higher risk of certain growth and developmental problems often termed congenital malformations.

Possible complications

If gestational diabetes is not managed properly, or goes undetected, it could cause a range of serious complications for both you and your baby, including:

- baby being large for its gestational age – i.e. weighing more than 4 kilos (8.8 pounds), known as macrosomia. This increases the need for induced labour or a caesarean birth, and may lead to birth problems such as shoulder dystocia;
- **premature birth** (your baby being born before week 37 of the pregnancy) – which can lead to complications such as newborn jaundice or respiratory distress syndrome;
- your baby having health problems shortly after birth that require hospital care – such as low blood sugar;
- miscarriage – the loss of a pregnancy during the first 23 weeks;
- stillbirth – the death of your baby around the time of the birth;
- shoulder dystocia, a possible consequence of having a large baby. This is when your baby's head passes through your vagina, but its shoulder gets stuck behind your pelvic bone (the ring of bone that supports your hip bones). Shoulder dystocia can be dangerous, as your baby may not be able to breathe while he or she is stuck. It's estimated to affect 1 in 200 births.

What is the problem with a high BMI?

Body mass index (BMI) is the balance between your height and your weight. It is used to work out whether you are underweight, just right, overweight or obese. Your BMI will be calculated and recorded in your pregnancy notes. This is a useful measurement as a higher BMI can affect your health and the success of the pregnancy.

- BMI less than 19 means you are underweight;
- BMI 19–25 means you are a healthy weight;
- BMI more than 25 means you are overweight;
- BMI more than 30 means you are obese.

Having a higher BMI is linked to your risk of developing diabetes. If your BMI is greater than 30 it is usually recommended that you take folic acid supplements for the first 12 weeks of pregnancy, plus vitamin D tablets for the whole of the pregnancy and the time that you are breastfeeding.

Other issues relating to a high BMI include:

- high blood pressure, pre-eclampsia
- more frequent urinary tract infections
- blood clotting disorders
- pelvic joint pains.

Obesity can also cause problems during labour and post-delivery complications such as an increased risk of bleeding. Following pregnancy there is also an increased chance of having urinary incontinence (therefore make sure that you keep up with the pelvic floor exercises).

Is there a silver lining to the cloud of being diagnosed with GDM?

If you think of gestational diabetes as being like a 'stress test' on your metabolism, then it is in principle showing you that you are at risk of developing metabolic problems later in life as the various risk factors and genetic predispositions will give you a higher chance of type 2 diabetes further down the line.

The diagnosis of GDM can for many act as an early warning shot and provide the opportunity to re-evaluate and adapt your approach to food and nutrition and your overall health – and this can even extend to your wider family. The start of your own self-management of GDM is an understanding of how best you can modify your diet and your attitude to food and exercise. Therefore, a lot is expected of you in terms of making sure that you look after yourself, dealing with the emotional stress of the diagnosis, starting to learn more about carbohydrates and the nutritional information on food packages and later on the possibility of medication or insulin injections.

One lovely side effect is that you get more scans to see baby, more chances to ask questions and meet the people who will care for you. Continuity of care is much more likely.

Getting ready to see the diabetes team – what do I need to know?

Your first appointment with your educator or dietician might only be 30 minutes long. During this time your dietician will want to do the following:

- explain to you the basics of GDM and your new diet;
- give you a blood glucose level testing machine, show you how to use it and record your results;
- give you some information about how to manage your carbohydrate intake (and what foods contain carbohydrates);
- tell you more about the risks involved with GDM and the importance of looking after yourself during pregnancy.

I don't understand a lot of what has been said!

Your educator or midwife or diabetes nurse has a lot of information to cover in that first appointment. But if you don't understand or you're confused you might be focusing on gathering the courage to interrupt them instead of hearing what is being said. Ask them to repeat things or explain it in a different way. Don't feel silly, pressured or out of time. This is your health and the wellbeing of your baby that is in question. Only you can make this experience what you want it to be.

3

Antenatal care – being supported during pregnancy

After a while, and having talked things through with Jon, Claire the midwife, her GP and her mum, Elizabeth realized that things were not as bad as she had first thought. Pregnancy is generally a lot safer now than ever before and with the right surveillance and support being available during the rest of her pregnancy she realized that she was not alone and that there were plenty of people out there to help her.

It still took a while to think of herself as having diabetes, as the only understanding she had of this before was what she'd seen in magazines with pictures of overweight people or stories of young children who had to inject themselves with insulin. Claire explained that gestational diabetes was a different form of the condition and arranged for her to be seen in the next few days at the local hospital.

In the obstetric department she met Hannah the midwife, who had special experience working with women with diabetes during pregnancy, and then she went across to the diabetes out-patient department where she met Julia, the diabetes specialist nurse, and Kirsty, the diabetes dietician. They had invited her to a group session for an introduction to gestational diabetes but Elizabeth told them she was rather nervous so they were able to meet for a one-on-one chat instead. They took the time to give her some background information on gestational diabetes, discussed some dietary issues about healthy eating and gave Elizabeth her own blood glucose meter, so that she could start testing her blood sugar levels. Elizabeth hadn't realized that she would need to regularly prick her fingers to produce droplets of blood for testing but decided that she was going to get on with it and not let this get in her way. She went home much more confident and better prepared.

What type of care should I expect?

The recognized, modern approach for women diagnosed with GDM is to have a form of shared care or multi-disciplinary team care which is designed to cover all the right needs during pregnancy.

First, your midwife may hand over or start to share your care with a dedicated diabetes midwife who will have special experience and training in helping to manage women with diabetes during pregnancy. You will also get to meet your local diabetes team which should consist of a diabetes specialist nurse (which is very different from the practice nurse in the local GP surgery), the consultant diabetologist (who is a doctor specifically trained in looking after people with diabetes – often with a specialist interest in diabetes in pregnancy) and a diabetes dietician (more on the importance of diet in GDM further on), and a consultant obstetrician with an interest in maternal medicine. Sometimes you may see some doctors in training, such as registrars, but these doctors will always be supervised by the specialists overseeing your care.

Your care should all take place under the auspices of an antenatal diabetes clinic and given the relatively short time period available to get things right and monitor you successfully, it may be that you are seen in this clinic every 2 weeks during your pregnancy. If you are still working then this can be a big commitment and inconvenience, but the majority of employers will be sympathetic to your needs and it is best to view your visits to the antenatal clinic as not one clinic appointment, but 3 or 4 consultations in one as you will see several members of the team each time you come.

Arriving at that first appointment with some questions ready to ask is going to help you feel prepared and in control. There is a lot to know once you get started. It helps to focus that first appointment on questions that are about getting you through the first week or two. Be sure to keep a note of other questions as they come up, either on your phone or in a notebook.

How often will I be seen and who by?

The care of the pregnant woman with diabetes is complex and it requires specialist knowledge.

Table 3.1 Recommended antenatal diabetes visit schedule

Appointment	The antenatal care that your team should offer
Booking appointment – ideally by 10 weeks of pregnancy	Test for GDM if you have had it before and are booking in the first 13 weeks
	Advice, information, support and treatment if you are diagnosed with GDM
12 weeks	Standard viability ultrasound scan
16 weeks	Test for GDM if you have had it before and are booking after 13 weeks
	Advice, information, support and treatment if you are diagnosed
20 weeks	20-week ultrasound scan to confirm that your baby is developing normally, including checks on baby's heart
24–28 weeks	Test for GDM if you haven't had it before but are at high risk of developing it
	Women diagnosed at this stage of pregnancy with GDM enter the pathway
	Advice, information, support and treatment if you are newly diagnosed
	Discuss information, education and advice about how diabetes will affect the pregnancy, birth and early parenting (such as breastfeeding and initial care of the baby)
28 weeks	Ultrasound scan to check your baby's growth
32 weeks	Ultrasound scan to check your baby's growth
	If this is your first baby, routine antenatal care that would be given at 31 weeks
36 weeks	Ultrasound scan
	Information and advice about:
	• planning the birth, including timing and types of birth, pain relief, and changes to your medications • changes to your treatments for diabetes during and straight after the birth • looking after your baby after birth, including starting breastfeeding and the effects of breastfeeding on your blood glucose • follow-up care and contraception

Appointment	The antenatal care that your team should offer
38 weeks	Tests to check your baby's wellbeing
	Advise you to have your labour induced, or a caesarean section if this is the best option, before 40 weeks if there are complications
39 weeks	Tests to check your baby's wellbeing
	Advise you to have your labour induced, or a caesarean section if this is the best option, before 41 weeks if you haven't had your baby by then

Source Adapted from NICE

The standard of care for patients with GDM is to be reviewed every 2 weeks in an antenatal clinic (Table 3.1). It is important to be seen regularly and most clinics are set up to be a 'one stop shop' in which you get to see everyone involved in your care. You may not see every team member each time – and be prepared to be seen by different people as over the course of your pregnancy team members may be working different shift patterns, e.g. working overnight delivering babies, going on study leave or being on-call. It may also be that you see trainee doctors and staff members working in each of the specialties, such as an obstetric registrar. Most antenatal clinics have a dedicated set of notes (which you should hold on to, as you are the most important person) in which everybody writes and which contains the plan for your care. This should (hopefully) be clear. Keep a list of who each of the team members are (there is normally space for this at the front of your notes) along with telephone numbers of who to call when there is a problem in between clinic visits.

What does the diabetes team do?

The diabetes team usually consists of the diabetes specialist nurse (DSN) and the diabetes consultant. They are mainly responsible for looking after the medical aspects of your care when it comes to treating things such as high blood pressure and glucose levels. They will be interested in making sure that you understand the implications of diabetes in pregnancy and supporting you in making diet and lifestyle changes to help improve your blood sugar levels.

They will provide advice about setting the right blood glucose targets for you based on your circumstances, understanding your risk factors for GDM and your future risk of having diabetes after pregnancy. The diabetes team will also be able to review the blood glucose monitoring results with you by going through the information that you have collected in your diary. They'll then be able to advise you on the right treatments at each stage of pregnancy and other factors such as baby's growth.

The DSN will usually act as your main point of contact and it is generally the case that the DSN is the person to call, email or leave messages with in between clinic visits.

What does the obstetrician do?

Obstetricians are doctors who specifically train in the field of women's health and have experience in looking after people during pregnancy, ensuring that any complications are treated; when the time comes, they can help plan and deliver baby. Your obstetrician will be interested in following you throughout the pregnancy and, working with the diabetologist, will be keen to ensure that your blood glucose levels are stable. If any problems arise during the pregnancy with either mother or baby then your obstetrician will know what to do and will explain the various treatment options and the best way of proceeding. Your obstetrician will be experienced in undertaking and interpreting ultrasound scans of the baby. Often, using the information from several growth scans performed over time, he or she can assess how well baby is doing by looking at the size of baby, baby's estimated weight and the amount of fluid around baby.

Towards the end of pregnancy your obstetrician will be able to talk to you about the best timing for delivery and taking into account your wishes, the best way of getting baby out.

What does the midwife do?

Midwives are the key professional in all pregnancies and births. The Department of Health policy document 'Maternity Matters: Choice, access and continuity of care' (2007) highlights the need for women to receive high quality safe care from a midwife:

> The benefits from improved outcomes for women and their babies are enhanced where care is specifically designed and deliv-

ered to meet the complex needs of women who have or who may develop diabetes.

The midwife's role is to support, advise and monitor the pregnant mum's health and wellbeing during her pregnancy and birth and to guide her and her family on the care of the newborn baby. Following enhanced education, training and experience, a midwife with an interest in diabetes care is best placed to provide support and guidance to a mother and her family where her care becomes increasingly complex. The midwife's role will be firmly embedded in the diabetes care pathway and this clearly recognizes the need for the enhancement of normal midwifery practice.

The midwife's role is also to enhance the normalization of the pregnancy, birth and postnatal experience for the woman and her baby; to provide education for women tailored to their specific individual needs, helping with self-care skills and support as well as reviewing care plans to aid women with diabetes prepare for a safe pregnancy.

What does the dietician do?

Food intake, portion control and diet type are all very important and relevant for controlling gestational diabetes. This is perhaps the most useful treatment intervention of all as the changes made in pregnancy can reap both immediate benefits and long-term gains.

The dietician in the antenatal clinic will have been specifically trained to know about both diabetes and the complexities of pregnancy. Your dietitian may ask you to keep a food diary before visits and it is often interesting to see the association between various food types and the impact they have on blood sugar levels.

The dietician will be able to talk to you about healthy eating options and making the right food choices during pregnancy (and beyond). It is often useful for you to meet her with your partner or other family members as the changes you may have to make won't be taking place in isolation. It would be odd (and unfair on you) to be having a different diet to the rest of your family (especially if you are the one doing the cooking). The recommendations that the dietician will make will take into account your own preferences and this is very important given the deeply personal relationship we often have with food, our likes and dislikes. I personally don't like any food that is coloured red.

The benefits of seeing the dietician are significant and the support that your dietician is able to provide can have lasting effects, especially in terms of improving your understanding of the impact of diet on your health, helping to shape behaviours relating to food, aiding weight loss and reducing the risk of getting diabetes later in life.

How will the baby be monitored during pregnancy?

Depending on the timing of your diagnosis, there should be a clear schedule of visits setting out what is going to happen on each occasion. The standard approach during any pregnancy is to have what is called a viability scan at 12 weeks gestation (to make sure that the pregnancy is established and developing in the right way), followed by a growth scan at 20 weeks to make sure that baby's growth is on track.

Given the importance of checking the growth of baby and looking for any congenital abnormalities, most antenatal clinics will have a set system of organizing a series of growth scans so that the pattern of baby's growth can be plotted and looked at on a chart of standardized growth measurements. Leg length and total body length are recorded and one of the key measures from the GDM perspective is that of how big baby's tummy is getting (the abdominal circumference or AC), as this is the position from which babies exposed to too much glucose can be prone to growing excessively. The trend of these measurements will be looked at over time to check on progress and will be reviewed regularly. Scanning may take place every 2 to 4 weeks depending on the centre, but don't necessarily expect a scan on every visit as extra scanning won't provide much more information.

Figure 3.1 shows the standard trajectory of baby growth during pregnancy (marked by the Xs). The gestational age is plotted along the bottom and the height of the fundus (the top of your bump) is plotted up the left hand side. The dark lines represent the upper and lower limits of normal growth patterns.

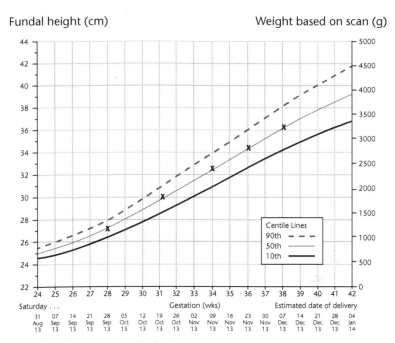

Figure 3.1 **Baby's growth during pregnancy**

The other test which is used in most antenatal clinics now is a dedicated ultrasound scan of baby's heart. This is one of the target organs which is at risk of not developing properly due to diabetes. This scan generally takes place around 22 weeks if you have pre-existing diabetes and may have to be done in a larger regional centre because of the specialized expertise required to perform such a technically difficult scan.

Why do I have to monitor my blood glucose levels?

Regular blood glucose monitoring can be painful and annoying. It is performed using a small digital device called a **glucometer**. There are several different types but all work on the general principle of having to insert a glucose test strip into the machine to activate it. Then, using some form of sharp lancet, you will have to stab the tip of one of your fingers (spring-loaded devices make this much easier) and produce a droplet of fresh blood – sometimes 'milking' the fingertip is required to get enough out – which can then be placed onto the waiting test strip. After 5 seconds or so the glucometer gives you a number (which in the UK is in the units of millimoles per litre (mmol/l) – in other parts of the world a different scale is used with units of grams per decilitre (g/dl)) that represents your blood glucose level at that time. A rough idea of the normal range for blood glucose levels is around 4 to 8 mmol/l in the non-pregnant state – and the body is usually very good at keeping glucose levels within these limits. Pregnancy naturally has a tendency to lower blood glucose values as there are several different physiological changes, including an increase in the amount of plasma (fluid) within the bloodstream, which will cause a degree of dilution.

Your antenatal diabetes nurse specialist or doctor will show you how to use the machine and advise on how often he or she will want you to test and record (often in a handy little glucose diary or booklet) your blood glucose values; this may be several times a day – before and after food – so that we can see the pattern of what is happening. You should have the target blood glucose values explained to you so that you know what to aim for in the fasting (before a meal) and the fed (post-meal) state.

There has been a lot of work done on how the day-to-day changes in the levels of glucose in the bloodstream affect mother and baby's health during pregnancy. Without an awareness of how glucose levels change, for example in response to certain foods and activities, it can be very difficult to understand what is happening and whether any glucose lowering treatments or dietary changes are needed. If for example the ultrasound scans during pregnancy show that there is an increase in baby's weight or size greater than expected it will be important to focus on blood glucose control and make decisions on treatment to get the levels into the target range. It is clearly better to be proactive and avoid this situation by having as good a level of blood glucose control as possible.

How do I test my blood sugars?

- Wash your hands in warm water. Don't use wet wipes as they contain glycerine, which could alter the result.

- Make sure your hands are warm. If they are really cold, it's hard to draw blood and finger pricking will hurt more.
- Prick the side of a finger. Avoid using your index finger or thumb as this can hurt more, and don't prick the middle or too close to a nail, because this can really hurt.
- Use a different finger each time and a different part of the finger. This will hurt less and help you to heal up.
- Keep a diary of your results. This will help your diabetes health-care team suggest any changes to your treatment, if needed.

How many times a day will I have to prick my finger?

If you consider that you need to know the fasting and post-meal values, then that will generally be 6 times per day (before and after breakfast, lunch and evening meal); a check before bedtime is also often recommended. In addition, extra checking may be required if there is a concern that blood sugar levels may be particularly high or low. Often after you have been doing this for the first few days, it becomes less painful and part of your normal routine. The most important thing is to make sure that you have been prescribed enough test strips to last you and if you run out don't wait until the next clinic appointment to get some more. Sometimes your GP may be reluctant to prescribe so many test strips (as it has to come out of their budget) but national guidance is clear about the necessity for regular, frequent testing and the relationship to better pregnancy outcomes. Any problems, speak to your midwife or diabetes nurse specialist.

Once it is clear that the glucose levels are stable, then the team may suggest that the frequency of blood monitoring can be dropped down. Sometimes people just check every other day, or just do one day with before-meal values and one day with after-meal readings.

What are the targets for blood sugar control?

This, so to speak, is a moveable feast depending on whereabouts you are receiving treatment. Generally before a meal the blood glucose values should be around 5.0 mmol/l or less and when checked again (1 hour after starting eating) the glucose level should be 7.0 mmol/l or lower.

These values may appear to be rather strict and difficult to achieve and different centres will have slightly different values. At the John Radcliffe Hospital in Oxford for example, doctors suggest 6.0 mmol/l as a fasting value and allow 7.8 mmol/l following a meal. These may be more realistic and easier to achieve. Some clinics even do 2-hour post-meal checking. If you are unable to test until 2 hours (rather than 1 hour) after a meal, the target level at that time should be below 6.4 mmol/l.

If you end up on insulin treatment or a tablet called glibenclamide to help manage your diabetes, the advice is to keep your glucose levels above 4.0 mmol/l because of the risks of **hypoglycaemia**.

The recently published NICE guidelines have tried to clarify these target levels and other international bodies such as the WHO also have their own recommendations. The aim however should not be to get too hung up on absolute values, but to take more stock of the general trend of the blood glucose values in order to get a feel for how stable the blood glucose control is overall.

It can often be tricky for both patients and clinicians to avoid an obsessiveness regarding blood glucose checking and a common-sense or pragmatic approach is usually required to maintain sanity. One may, for example, become stressed over a few overly high glucose values following a meal out with friends or a Sunday roast when the rest of the time the glucose values are in the target range and follow a nice pattern. The assessment that too many glucose values are out of target and likely to cause a problem roughly relates to whether 50 per cent or more of the readings at a particular time of day, e.g. after breakfast, are out of target (see below). We do know that persistently high blood glucose values or highly variable levels are associated with the complications of diabetic pregnancy that we wish to avoid.

The glucose diary shown in Table 3.2 demonstrates a common clinical scenario, where most of the glucose levels are at a satisfactory level but a few are out of kilter. This is perhaps because of eating too much or having the wrong type of carbohydrate. Or potentially too much physical activity which can increase the consumption of blood glucose and consequently cause low blood glucose readings. By looking through the record of your changing daily glucose values it is possible to work with your healthcare

Table 3.2 Glucose diary

	Before breakfast	1 hour after breakfast	Before lunch	1 hour after lunch	Before dinner	1 hour after dinner	Before bedtime
Monday	4.5	7.9	3.5	6.7	4.7	9.4	8.3
Tuesday	5.1	8.5		5.9	5.0	10.2	
Wednesday			2.5	6.0	4.1	7.4	9.1
Thursday	3.8	8.0	11.1	5.8	5.0	7.9	
Friday	4.4	8.1	4.4	6.1	3.3	9.1	7.8
Saturday	4.8		4.9		4.4	10.2	
Sunday		9.6	5.2	7.8	3.9	7.7	

providers and understand what is working well (perhaps having porridge for breakfast) and what is adversely affecting you (you may need a snack to keep your glucose levels up when walking home from work in the afternoon). Don't forget your diary when you come to the antenatal clinic!

Why won't my GP prescribe me enough test strips?

The latest NICE guidance now makes it clear how frequently blood glucose testing should be done. It is not uncommon to see patients who complain about not being able to get enough test strips prescribed for all the testing that they need to be doing during pregnancy. If you have any difficulties getting hold of the right amount of test strips to do the right amount of glucose testing, then the diabetes team or your midwife can get in contact with your GP to advise them and remember all of your prescriptions should be free during pregnancy.

Why can't I have a continuous glucose monitor rather than having to repeatedly stab myself?

Ever since the introduction of blood glucose testing, specialists have been trying to come up with a way in which to overcome the frustrating problems of multiple daily blood glucose tests. One system which has been around for a few years now is called the continuous glucose monitoring system (CGMS). This involves the insertion of a small plastic tube or cannula through the skin (usually on the stomach) down into the fatty tissues below. The tube is attached to an electronic sensor which sits on the abdominal wall and records the glucose level in the fatty tissues on a continuous basis. The sensor sits there for several days before being taken off and the data analysed. Now, unfortunately, such CGMS systems are not commonly used in the context of GDM because they don't tend to add much extra to the information that you get from normal, regular self-monitoring of blood glucose. They can also be cumbersome (and are expensive for the NHS as they are not routinely funded at the time of writing). They are generally reserved for patients with pre-existing type 1 diabetes who are already on multiple daily injections of insulin with very difficult-to-manage blood glucose levels. You may come across fellow patients in the antenatal diabetes clinic who are attached to CGMS sensors, or even insulin pump devices, but there are presently very few (i.e. nil) places that would use a CGMS system for an individual with GDM.

What about very low blood sugars?

Hypoglycaemia (hypos) is the name given to low blood sugars. There is no universally agreed definition but essentially it relates to having a low recorded blood sugar level of around 3.5 mmol/l or less (it differs for different people – some being more or less sensitive), along with symptoms such as:

- trembling or shakiness
- sweating
- anxiety or irritability
- turning pale
- feeling hungry.

You may be at risk of hypoglycaemia if you are using glibenclamide or insulin injections to control your gestational diabetes.

Learn the risks of hypoglycaemia, and learn how to recognize the effects. If hypoglycaemia is not treated it may lead to unconsciousness, because there is not enough glucose for the brain to function normally. The immediate treatment of hypoglycaemia is to have some sugary food or drink, such as Lucozade, glucose or dextrose tablets and unsweetened fruit juice. You may be given a concentrated glucose drink to keep on hand in case you have hypoglycaemia. One difficult-to-master trick is then not to overdo the treatment and neck every bottle of Lucozade in sight. Hypoglycaemia is not a nice sensation and the temptation is to take on board lots of carbohydrate, but this then makes things shoot the other way with hyperglycaemia and can take a while to sort out!

I can't get it right!

Don't worry. It's difficult. You've suddenly got a whole new medical problem to deal with and it can be tricky to get to grips with. One of the main issues is that it is so linked to lifestyle and what we do every day that there is a huge amount of guilt and blame surrounding GDM – as though this has been deliberately brought on by yourself!

Nobody will expect your blood glucose levels to be perfect straight away. This takes time and effort to achieve and you will have the support of all the team members in the antenatal clinic to help you. You will not be the first or last person to be frustrated by GDM, but it would be very surprising to find that you can't be helped. We talk a lot more about glucose, diet and getting on top of things later on in Chapters 4 to 8.

4

Diet and lifestyle – the cornerstones of gestational diabetes management

Elizabeth initially did not like the assumption that there was something wrong with the food that she had been eating. She had always prided herself on being a good cook and watched what she ate, as well as going for walks at weekends or going to aerobics after work. After talking with Kirsty, the diabetes dietician, it became apparent that actually there were no problems with her food and what she had been eating was a fairly standard healthy diet. Kirsty explained however that changes to the body during pregnancy, and the way in which the body handles glucose when gestational diabetes is present, mean that the body processes foods differently.

Kirsty was able to explain about the 'glycaemic index' and how some food types are absorbed much quicker than others – the difference in behaviour between cornflakes and Weetabix when they get into your body for example – and was able to provide all sorts of alternative suggestions for Elizabeth's diet that would allow her body to suffer fewer glucose surges and enjoy more stable blood sugar levels. Armed with meal plans and a list of healthy snacks, Elizabeth and Jon set off to the supermarket and were able to do their weekly shop with open minds and plenty of ideas.

Why is diet so important with gestational diabetes?

There are two main aspects to the human metabolism. First, what happens in the rested or fasted state – when the cells and tissues are ticking over minding their own business, using up fuel at a fairly steady rate of combustion. Second, there is the active part of our lives when we are busy and there are fluctuating demands on the fuel supply or there is a sudden influx of glucose entering our bodies from the gut.

Gestational diabetes relates to how the body handles glucose in both situations. In the rested scenario, the body is both consuming glucose and generating some of its own from its stores in the liver. Higher blood sugar levels under such circumstances relate to pre-determined metabolic and genetic factors, plus an element of insulin resistance. Little can be done to modify this aspect of things in the short term.

When we eat, however, all sorts of physiological cascades and hormonal activity are let loose, resulting in metabolic changes as glucose enters the body from the gut and hits the bloodstream. The speed at which it is absorbed and the amount of carbohydrate eaten are the key factors here and are eminently modifiable. Adjusting your dietary intake can have a big impact on blood glucose levels in GDM and significantly help to improve the situation. First stop – the diabetes dietician.

What will happen when I see the dietician?

The dietician will be very skilled at getting to understand you and your diet. Your dietician will be able to talk to you about the basics of gestational diabetes and the importance of eating regularly and how certain foods will impact on your blood glucose levels more than others.

Your dietician can go into some detail about your carbohydrate intake and how to manage this – and will give you an overview of which particular foods contain carbohydrates (and their behaviour). Your dietician will provide you in addition with some information about meal plans, the low GI diet and suitable snack options, as it is often difficult to know where to begin.

The general principle for eating for women with GDM is to go for three regular medium-sized meals per day, as well as three regular snacks between meals each day. This combination has been shown to help maintain blood glucose levels most effectively. Sometimes people may find it is difficult to eat like this or to take on board snacks when they don't feel particularly hungry. It may be that you are used to skipping breakfast or lunch or don't like the idea of eating when you are at work or in-between meals. It is always best to work with your dietician to find the best solution for you – rather than feel like you are being told what to do. Trial and error is often a sensible approach when you are getting started as we know everybody's metabolism (and lifestyle) is slightly different.

With so much to take in, you could still come away from appointments feeling unsure about the right answers. And there are lots of myths about diabetes and food that you will need to navigate, too. If you've just been diagnosed and aren't sure about what you can and can't eat, here's what you need to know.

Principles for dietary management of GDM

1 Careful with carbohydrates.
2 Go low GI (slow release carbs).
3 Reduce sugar.
4 Eat regularly.
5 Perfect portion sizes.
6 Avoid 'diabetic foods'.

What are carbohydrates?

Carbohydrates or carbs are an important part of any diet and are the main source of fuel or energy (and include sugars, starch and cellulose). The technical definition is that they are:

> any of a large group of organic compounds occurring in foods and living tissues. They contain hydrogen and oxygen in the same ratio as water (2:1) and typically can be broken down to release energy in the animal body.

Carbohydrates form the basis of the human diet along with the other major classes of nutrients: fat and protein.

Examples of carbohydrate-containing food include wheat, bread, rice, potatoes and couscous. When consumed they are digested, absorbed and converted into glucose (one of many types of sugar) which is then used by the body as a fuel supply for the tissues such as the muscles and brain. Carbohydrates are sucked up from the gut and travel in the bloodstream to where they are needed. The important hormone which controls this process is insulin (more on this later), which activates the uptake of glucose. The action of insulin in gestational diabetes is less effective than normal and this subsequently means that levels of glucose within the blood can rise and fluctuate depending on what and how much has been eaten. The excess glucose sloshing around inside the body is what we seek to avoid in GDM.

Food is not the only factor which impacts on blood glucose levels but it is an important one and relatively easy to modify.

Can't I just get rid of all carbohydrates from my diet? Can't I just carb restrict?

Given that we know that 'too much glucose is bad', the temptation might be to remove carbohydrates from the diet in order to overcome the problems of gestational diabetes. This however is not a good approach as several hundreds of thousands of years of human evolution have occurred to avoid your blood sugar levels dropping when you starve. In the carbohydrate restricted state, the human body will begin to think it is in starvation mode and activate various metabolic cascades to overcome the lack of fuel intake. This mainly consists of the breakdown of pre-existing glucose and fat stores and the production of new glucose by the liver. The triggering of these energy reserves causes marked surges or spikes in blood glucose levels – and we know that blood glucose variability is bad – while the breakdown of fat stores for energy production creates a substance called ketones – which are a good temporary fuel supply, but if this is prolonged they can build up. They are acidic and are not good for baby's brain and can make you feel lethargic, sick and cause headaches.

Simply cutting out carbohydrates means that you will not have adequate nutrient and glucose levels for your own energy requirements or enough fuel for baby's growth, and you run the risk of fluctuating blood sugar levels and potentially toxic effects on baby. What you ideally need to achieve is a level of regular and consistent carbohydrate consumption that your body is able to handle without causing high blood glucose levels.

What is the low GI diet?

Things get more complicated when we consider that not all carbo-hydrates are the same. The **glycaemic index** of carbohydrates essentially rates how quickly they are digested and absorbed into the bloodstream. Developed in 1982 at the University of Toronto, the glycaemic index (GI) is a system for comparing carbohydrates based on their effect on blood glucose levels. Foods which are 'high' GI, such as doughnuts for example, are very rapidly absorbed into the blood and cause blood sugar fluctuations. Low GI foods (whole-grain breads, basmati rice) are digested and enter the system far more slowly and as such give your body more time to respond with the insulin needed to process them.

The low GI diet plan is recommended because it will:

- prevent big fluctuations in blood sugar levels;
- make you feel fuller for longer and reduce your hunger;
- help you manage your weight;
- help reduce cholesterol;
- help to reduce insulin resistance.

The majority of GDM can be controlled through dietary measures, generally by eating smaller amounts of low GI food spaced out over the course of the day. This might work out roughly as:

- *breakfast*, 30 grams carbohydrates
- *mid-morning snack*, 15 grams carbohydrates
- *lunch*, 25–30 grams carbohydrates
- *mid-afternoon snack*, 15 grams carbohydrates
- *evening meal*, 45 grams carbohydrates
- *bedtime snack*, 15 grams carbohydrates.

This will be about 1,800 calories per day; in addition, as part of the balanced approach to diet, the amount of protein and fat will be about 60 grams each, plus around 25 grams of fibre per day. Carbohydrate counting is useful (but not essential) and will form part of the discussion with your dietician when learning what are the best things to eat (and what to avoid). If the carbohydrate intake is too high, then this can cause the blood glucose levels to rise up. Conversely, not enough carbohydrate can mean low blood sugars for you and not enough fuel for baby.

Eating well does take a bit of planning and sometimes you might need to get up a little earlier to make sure that you have the time to make a well-balanced breakfast. Try thinking about preparing meals in advance or batch cooking to make life easier.

What makes a food low or high GI?

This mostly depends on the relative proportion of amylose (one type of starch) to amylopectin (another type of starch) within the food. Foods that have a greater ratio of amylose, for example lentils, have a lower glycaemic index than foods with a relatively greater proportion of amylopectin, like potatoes, which have a high glycaemic index. Pure glucose or sugar, as the benchmark, has a GI score of 100 and is absorbed very quickly by the body and causes spikes in blood sugar levels.

If you typically eat a lot of processed food – breakfast cereals, white bread, biscuits and cakes (lots of refined, pure sugar) – there will be a lot of quickly available energy in your blood, and your metabolism will use this energy rather than turning to your own fat stores. More starchy foods with slow release carbohydrates, such as oats and wholegrain, do not have this dramatic effect. A low glycaemic index diet is therefore one that selects foods on the basis of minimal changes in circulating glucose levels (or low GI score; Table 4.1 overleaf).

Eating low GI carbohydrate foods causes a steady rise in the level of glucose in the blood, which in turn leads to a small and gentle rise in insulin. Small increases in insulin keep you feeling full and energized for hours after eating and also encourage the body to burn fat.

- Low GI foods provide natural, slowly released energy.
- Generally, the less processed a carbohydrate, the more likely it is to have a low GI score.
- Foods that are white, including processed foods made with white flour and white sugar, tend to have a high GI and cause a sudden surge in your blood sugars.
- High-fibre foods take longer to digest and therefore produce a slower rise in blood sugar levels. Fibre also keeps you feeling

Table 4.1 Glycaemic index of everyday foodstuffs

	Low GI foodstuffs GI below 55	Medium GI foodstuffs GI 55–70	High GI foodstuffs GI over 70
Breakfast cereals	Porridge (42) All-Bran (30) Natural muesli (40) Rolled oats (50)	Mini Wheats (58) Nutrigrain (66) Shredded Wheat (66) Special K (68)	Cornflakes (80) Puffed wheat (80) Cheerios (74) Rice Krispies (80) Weetabix (75) Sultana Bran (72) Bran Flakes (74) Coco Pops (77)
Bread	Wholegrain (46) Wholewheat (49) Sourdough wheat or rye (52) Soya and linseed (36)	Croissant (67) Hamburger bun (61) White pitta (57) Wholemeal rye (62)	White (71) Bagel (72) French baguette (95)
Dairy	Whole milk (30) Skimmed milk (31) Sweetened yoghurt (32) Soy milk (44) Custard (35) Chocolate milk (41)	Ice cream (62)	
Staples	New potatoes (54) White long grain rice (50) Brown rice (50) Pearl barley (23) Sweet potatoes (48) Instant noodles (45) Wheat pasta (54)	Basmati rice (58) Couscous (64) Canned potatoes (63) Baked potatoes (60) Wild rice (55)	Instant white rice (85) Short-grain white rice (84) Fresh mashed potatoes (75) Chips (75) Instant mashed potatoes (80)
Vegetables	Frozen peas (40) Frozen sweetcorn (45) Raw carrots (16) Boiled carrots (41) Aubergine (15) Broccoli (10) Cauliflower (15)	Beetroot (60)	Pumpkin (75) Parsnips (95)

	Low GI foodstuffs GI below 55	Medium GI foodstuffs GI 55–70	High GI foodstuffs GI over 70
Vegetables (continued)	Cabbage (10) Mushrooms (10) Tomatoes (14) Lettuce (10) Green beans (15) Bell peppers (10) Onions (10)		
Fruits	Cherries (22) Plums (24) Grapefruit (25) Peaches (28) Peaches, canned in juice (30) Apples (34) Pears (41) Dried apricots (32) Grapes (43) Kiwi fruit (47) Oranges (40) Strawberries (40) Prunes (29)	Mango (60) Sultanas (56) Bananas (58) Raisins (64) Pineapple (66)	Watermelon (80) Dates (100)
Legumes (Beans)	Kidney beans (52) Butter beans (36) Chickpeas (42) Haricot beans (31) Red lentils (21) Green lentils (30)	Beans in tomato sauce (56)	
Snacks	Snickers bar (41) Muesli bar (49) Sponge cake (46) Nutella (33) Milk chocolate (42) Hummous (6) Peanuts (13) Walnuts (15) Cashew nuts (25) Nuts and raisins (21) Jam (51)	Ryvita (63) Digestives (59) Blueberry muffin (59) Honey (58) Oatmeal crackers (55)	Water crackers (78) Rice cakes (87) Puffed crispbread (81) Doughnuts (76) Scones (92)

fuller for longer, which helps prevent overeating. Most vegetables, wholegrains, legumes, nuts, seeds and fruits are rich in fibre when you eat them whole.

To switch to a low GI diet

- Choose brown (wholegrain) versions of foods like bread, pasta, rice and crackers.
- Always combine protein like fish, chicken and dairy foods with carbs like bread, potatoes and pasta – for example, when snacking combine a handful of nuts (protein) with a piece of fruit (carbs).
- Use new potatoes instead of old and boil in their skins rather than mashing, baking or chipping.
- Thicken sauces using a little tahini or nut butter rather than high GI cornflour.
- Choose amylose-rich basmati rice instead of other varieties of white rice.
- Avoid 'instant' or 'easy cook' foods which tend to be more highly processed.
- Snack on unsalted nuts, seeds or oatcakes rather than sweet treats and biscuits.
- Include at least one low GI food with each meal and snack.
- Use vinegar and lemon juice dressings or sauces. The acidity lowers the GI of carbohydrates.
- Don't overcook carbohydrate type foods, this can increase the GI of carbohydrates.
- Include protein in your meals and snacks. Protein foods include lean meat, chicken, fish, egg, reduced fat cheese and legumes.
- Include peas, beans and lentils, for example baked beans, kidney beans, butter beans, chick peas. They contain both proteins and carbohydrates and are low in GI.
- Include lots of non-starchy vegetables and salads.

There is a meal plan and recipe ideas at the end of this chapter.

What are the health effects of eating a low GI diet in pregnancy?

A positive side effect is that you may lose weight following a low GI eating regime. That's because these sorts of foods tend to keep you feeling fuller for longer. Although it's worth remembering that low GI does not mean low fat, so you may need to watch the fat content of your meals.

A low GI eating plan can also be helpful if you're worried about your risk of type 2 diabetes and heart disease. A low GI diet improves blood sugar and insulin control and helps manage cholesterol levels. Stabilizing blood sugar levels should also mean that you feel improvements in energy, mood and concentration levels.

Breakfast ideas

- Weetabix
- All-Bran flakes
- Greek yoghurt with fruit
- Apple and linseed porridge
- Muesli with hazelnuts and raspberries (be careful with the type, however, as some muesli brands are packed with sugar to make them more tasty)
- Poached or scrambled eggs on wholemeal toast
- Grapefruit, apricot and orange salad
- Cinnamon granola bars
- 2-egg mushroom omelette with spinach
- Scrambled tofu with tomatoes
- Spelt flour pancakes with fruit and yoghurt
- Courgette and corn muffins
- Banana and blueberry low GI bread.

Here are some other breakfast foods rated by GI index:

- *Breakfast foods with a low GI index (below 55)*, cheese, eggs, hash browns, rolled oats, semi-skimmed milk, whole-wheat bread, mixed grain bread, oranges.
- *Breakfast foods with a medium GI index (55–70)*, bananas (but avoid very ripe bananas), bran and blueberry muffins, croissants, instant porridge or oatmeal, shredded wheat cereal, Special K.

- *Breakfast foods with a high GI index (more than 70)*, white bread, Cheerios, Rice Krispies, bagels, breakfast scones, waffles.

What about snacks?

Many centres recommend regular snacks throughout the day for people with diabetes during pregnancy, i.e. mid-morning, mid-afternoon and at bedtime. This helps to maintain stable blood glucose levels, keep hunger at bay, avoid hypoglycaemia and block your liver from releasing its own glucose stores. If you treat your diabetes with certain medications that put you at risk of hypoglycaemia, then snacks are helpful. However, if your medications are making you snack regularly to prevent hypos, speak to your healthcare team.

If you are getting hungry, choose healthy snacks such as fruit and vegetables. The key is to plan for these snacks, be mindful of your portion sizes and monitor their effect on your blood glucose levels. Limit your intake of calorie-rich, but nutritionally poor, snacks and drinks, such as sweets, cakes, crisps, fizzy drinks, energy drinks, etc.

Low GI snack examples

- Handful of almonds or walnuts
- Apple crisps
- Wholewheat crackers with peanut butter
- Seed mix (sunflower, linseeds and pumpkin seeds)
- Hummous with vegetables for dipping (cucumbers, peppers,
- Sweet potato wedges
- Toasted whole-wheat pitta bread
- Fresh soybeans with a pinch of salt
- One-third of a cup of dried apricots
- Rice cakes or oatcakes
- Hard boiled egg
- Sliced pear with goat's cheese
- Blueberries and raspberries with sunflower seeds
- Root vegetable crisps
- Greek yoghurt
- Granola bar
- One-quarter cup salsa with one-quarter cup cottage cheese and 10 tortilla chips

- 10 pretzels with 2 tablespoons peanut or almond butter
- 2 squares of dark chocolate (more than 70 per cent cocoa solids).

It may feel unusual to take regular snacks when you are not normally used to doing so. Snacking between meals is a useful way of helping to reduce hunger and can actively contribute to stabilizing your glucose levels and providing extra energy. Remember, snacks should only be eaten in moderation.

Lunch examples

Take a few minutes each evening to make your lunch and get it ready for the next day. That way, if you are running late the next morning, lunch is ready to go and you aren't forced to dine on vending machine rubbish.

- Tuna rainbow salad with wholegrain bread
- Fried rice with vegetables, cashew nuts and tofu
- Pasta with crushed garlic and salmon
- Wholemeal pitta bread with salad, yoghurt and tuna, egg or salmon
- Baked sweet potato with veggie filling
- Prawn and grapefruit noodle salad
- Green club sandwich
- Pea, courgette and pesto soup
- Tomato and pepper spicy soup
- Mexican bean salad
- Lamb steaks with barley
- Baked beans on wholemeal toast
- Sliced chicken breast wrap with sweetcorn, low-fat dressing and raw salad
- Avocado dip with raw vegetables
- Cottage cheese and salad sandwiches.

Dinner examples

- Noodles with stir-fried beef
- Macaroni and kidney bean salad
- Barbecued sesame beef with red cabbage and coleslaw
- Spiced chicken stew
- Sea bass with lemon and fennel

- Chicken and mushroom risotto
- Lean minced beef and sweet potato stew
- Salmon and broccoli tray bake
- Garlic prawns and lentils
- Whole-wheat pasta, almonds and broccoli
- Chickpea curry
- Chilli chicken soup
- Beef and pot barley
- Mixed rice, beans and chorizo
- Quinoa, chicken and pumpkin soup
- Lamb chops and Greek salad
- Couscous and chickpea salad
- Roast lamb with roasted vegetables
- Chicken and herb meatballs
- Chicken and bean enchiladas.

But low GI food is boring. There's too much food I miss. What can I do?

Low GI foods will be digested more slowly than medium and high GI foods so you will feel full for longer and will be able to eat fewer calories without feeling hungry. It is also worth noting that adding a low GI food to a meal will lower the glycaemic index of the whole meal.

Foods to avoid

We try not to be food zealots, but it is clear that there are certain foods which even in moderation can cause problems with your metabolism and we recommend avoiding them altogether during pregnancy. Many people find that the changes in diet that they make following a diagnosis of GDM help change both their short-term and long-term eating habits and help to get rid of a sweet tooth. Any such dietary changes are best done by the whole family, as having a healthy meal can be very difficult when sitting next to someone drinking coke and eating a plate of pizza. This also means not adding sugar or sweeteners to food, including honey. Foods to avoid include:

- Processed breakfast products such as cornflakes, pastries, bagels, doughnuts, sugary breakfast cereals.
- Fizzy drinks. There are 9 teaspoons of sugar in a can of coke – need I say more?
- Pork, sausage rolls, lamb, hot dogs and beef, all of which are high GI. Instead eat chicken, turkey, white fish and shellfish. Beans are a healthy meat alternative and most are low GI, including kidney beans, lentils and black-eyed peas.
- Carbohydrates that have lots of added sugar or honey that are made from refined white flour, and foods with lots of added fat. Some examples include cakes, croissants, puddings, sweet biscuits, pastry, juice, soft drinks, cordials, lollies, chips, pizza, fried foods and takeaway food.

Someone has just bought me some diabetic food from the supermarket. What should I do?

Avoid foods labelled 'diabetic' or 'suitable for diabetics'. These foods contain similar amounts of calories and fat to non-diabetic foods, and they can affect your blood glucose levels. They are usually more expensive and can have a laxative effect. Stick to your usual foods. If you want to have an occasional treat, go for what you would have normally and keep an eye on your portions.

Is there anything else I should avoid eating while pregnant?

Avoid fish which tend to have higher levels of mercury, e.g. tuna. It is also advisable to avoid raw shellfish to reduce the risk of getting food poisoning, which can be particularly unpleasant. Avoid certain types of cheese, raw or uncooked eggs and meat, liver and unpasteurized milk.

What about alcohol?

There is controversy and uncertainty about the safety of alcohol in pregnancy. And the honest answer is not clear. Certainly, heavy drinking is not a good idea. Perhaps the safest option is not to drink alcohol at all while you're pregnant. It is particularly important to avoid alcohol during the first three months of pregnancy as alcohol may be associated with an increased risk of miscarriage.

We all know that binge drinking is not good for our health. For pregnant women, getting drunk, or binge drinking (defined as drinking more than 7.5 units of alcohol on a single occasion) can be harmful to the unborn baby. Alcohol can also make hypoglycaemia more likely to occur if you treat your gestational diabetes with insulin or glibenclamide.

I want to avoid becoming overweight

Pregnancy isn't the time to be on a really strict diet. I suggest that you don't aim to lose weight while you're pregnant – this could be unsafe for you and your baby. However, small changes to your diet and physical activity levels can help you to avoid gaining excess weight during your pregnancy. This will help you to manage your gestational diabetes better and increase your chances of having a healthy pregnancy.

People with gestational diabetes are at a high risk of getting the condition again in subsequent pregnancies as well as getting type 2 diabetes in the future. Therefore, it is very important to continue your healthy eating plan after having your baby in order to manage your weight and reduce your risk of developing gestational diabetes in subsequent pregnancies, as well as your long-term risk of getting type 2 diabetes.

If I can't control my blood glucose overnight shouldn't I just cut out carbs after lunchtime?

No, that won't help. If you are waking with higher than recommended glucose levels then this is due to your liver releasing glucose overnight, which isn't improved by reducing your dietary carbohydrate. If this is the case, further treatment is needed. This may be tablets or insulin depending on your treating centre.

Don't skip meals

Try to eat balanced meals at regular intervals each day and have the same amount of food at each one. Eat three small to moderate-sized meals every day. Using a smaller dinner plate can help you keep an eye on your portion sizes. You can also eat between two and four snacks, including an after-dinner snack to help keep your blood sugar levels steady.

What about fat?

Fats have a pretty bad reputation but we do need them. They help with insulating our organs and regulating our body temperature, and aid the absorption of fat-soluble vitamins (A, D, E and K).

How do fats work in my body?

Like protein, fat doesn't turn into glucose but there does seem to be some indirect effect on blood glucose levels with some higher fat foods. Saturated (or animal) fat tends to make it harder for your insulin to work (similar to how your placental hormones do) and so if you have a creamy sauce on a pasta or eat a pie or a croissant, you will often see a higher glucose level after you eat because the fat has made it more difficult to clear the glucose from the carbohydrate also included in those foods.

What are the best fats to eat while I am pregnant?

Eating too much fat when you are pregnant makes it easy to gain excess weight, and if you are eating a lot of saturated fat (full-cream dairy, fatty meats, snacks such as muffins, chips or biscuits) these can cause excessively high cholesterol that can also accelerate your baby's growth – especially when you have gestational diabetes. Fats can interfere with the way in which your body processes glucose and the effects can last for many hours after a meal. Try to avoid deep-fried foods and takeaways such as chips, burgers and pizzas.

The healthiest fat choices are olive oil and other vegetable oils (except palm), avocado, nuts, oily fish and lean meats.

Troubleshooting

If your glucose readings are high after eating a meal, consider the following.

- Try reducing the overall amount of carbohydrates in the meal by one-quarter and see if this makes a difference.
- Aim to spread your carbohydrate intake over the course of the whole day. Could you have a smaller meal and a snack later on?
- Make sure that your meals are balanced with proteins and non-starchy vegetables. Carbs should not dominate.
- Was the meal high in fat?

I've changed my diet, I've been walking every day and doing all the right things, but my blood sugar levels just keep on going up. What am I doing wrong?

Probably nothing. One of the infuriating things about GDM is that you can't always predict how things are going to go. It is possible to make sensible dietary changes and yet still have hyperglycaemia. This is not your fault, it's not baby's fault, it's not anybody's fault, this frankly is just the nature of gestational diabetes – an impaired ability of your body to produce enough insulin to control the glucose. This is the time when we need to think about other ways to get the sugar levels under control – see Chapters 5 and 6.

Meal plan

It's important to mix up the example meals in the meal plan (see Table 4.2) as eating the same things every day can get boring. The effects on your blood sugar will become apparent through trial and error.

Table 4.2 Weekly meal plan example

	Breakfast	Mid-morning	Lunch	Mid-afternoon	Evening meal	Bedtime
Monday	2 x wholegrain toast with peanut butter	1 x apple	Pitta bread with tuna salad	Handful of grapes	Spicy chicken stew	Seedmix
Tuesday	Porridge	Handful of almonds	Quick pasta with lamb	Handful of almonds	Quinoa, chicken and pumpkin soup	Toasted wholemeal pitta bread
Wednesday	Scrambled eggs on toast	Dried apricots	Chicken salad wrap	Hard boiled egg	Chickpea curry	Granola bar
Thursday	Weetabix with sliced bananas	Seed and nut mix	Tomato soup	1 x peach	Stir fried beef and noodles	Sliced pear with goat's cheese
Friday	Porridge	1 x pear	Baked beans on wholemeal toast	Wholewheat crackers	Mixed rice, beans and chorizo	2 squares of dark chocolate
Saturday	Greek yoghurt with blueberries	3 x oatcakes with peanut butter	Greek salad with prawns	Raisin toast and glass of milk	Garlic prawns and lentils	1 x apple
Sunday	Spelt pancakes with raspberries and strawberries	Vegetable crisps	Roasted lamb with roasted vegetables	Oatmeal biscuits x 2	Chicken and herb meatballs	2 x oatcakes

Low GI recipes

Black Bean Scramble (serves two)

This is a healthy breakfast idea with plenty of protein, good fats from the avocado and the olive oil as well as greenery with the spinach.

Ingredients

- 4 medium eggs
- Seasoning spices such as cumin seeds, cayenne pepper plus 1 clove of crushed garlic
- Olive oil
- 1 small onion, chopped
- 1 tin black beans, drained
- 1 medium tomato, diced
- Handful of fresh spinach, chopped
- 1 avocado (ensure ripe), chopped
- 1 grapefruit, halved.

Method

1 Mix the eggs and spices together.
2 Heat the olive oil in a frying pan and gently cook the onion until soft.
3 Pour over the egg mixture.
4 Throw in the drained tin of black beans and the chopped tomato.
5 Then add the chopped spinach and cook until the eggs are done to your liking.
6 Divide into two portions and then add the chopped avocado.
7 Serve with the grapefruit halves.

Cereal mix with fresh fruit (serves two)

Having a pear with a mixture of seeds and nuts gives you a low GI fruit load, while flax meal contains plenty of omega 3 oil and has a nice nutty flavour.

Ingredients

- 2 tbsp flax meal

- 2 tbsp sesame seeds
- 2 tbsp almond meal
- 2 tbsp hazelnut meal
- ½ tsp vanilla
- ½ tsp cinnamon
- 1 cup of plain Greek yoghurt
- Sliced pear

Method

1 Place the first six ingredients in a medium-sized mixing bowl and stir together.
2 Split the mixture into two bowls and then top with the yoghurt and sliced pear.

Butternut squash and poached eggs (serves two)

A well-balanced tasty meal that can be eaten at any time of day. It also has the benefit of being gluten free.

Ingredients

- Olive oil
- 1 butternut squash, chopped
- ½ courgette, chopped
- 1 small red onion, chopped
- 2 tsp curry powder
- ½ tsp cinnamon
- 1 or 2 eggs

Method

1 Heat the olive oil in a medium to large frying pan.
2 Throw the vegetables, curry powder, cinnamon and a pinch of salt into the pan.
3 Cook through and stir until the pieces of squash are beginning to get brown and crisp.
4 Then start to poach two eggs in a pan of boiling water.
5 When the squash is soft or tender take off the heat.
6 Drain the eggs and serve together with the vegetable mixture, season to your taste.

Spinach frittata bites (serves two)

A healthy, easy cook savoury snack that goes well with a green salad. You'll need a muffin tray with 6 or 8 holes for this recipe.

Ingredients

- 1 small red onion, chopped
- Olive oil
- Frozen spinach, approx. 10 grams, defrosted and squeezed dry
- 2 cloves of garlic
- 6 large eggs
- Salt, pepper, nutmeg

Method

1 Preheat the oven to 350 degrees Celsius.
2 Grease the inside of an 8-hole muffin tray with olive oil.
3 In a small frying pan, heat the rest of the olive oil and cook the chopped onion until soft.
4 Stir in the crushed garlic and spinach for about a minute, then set to one side.
5 Whisk together the eggs and seasoning and then pour over the vegetable mixture.
6 Stir this all together and then divide equally between the muffin cups.
7 Bake for about 15 minutes until enlarged and nicely browned.
8 Remove from the tray and serve while still warm.

What is recommended for my future diet?

A healthy, balanced diet – that means eating regular meals, choosing good sources of carbohydrates and watching your portions, including fruit and vegetables, and eating less saturated fat, sugar and salt.

5

Now you're telling me that I have to exercise?!

Elizabeth was struggling with the diet changes because there were lots of things that she missed and really wanted. Sometimes she went off-track and ate some 'banned' food off someone else's plate.

Overall, her glucose levels were certainly better, but often after a meal (especially in the evenings) they were just creeping over the target and she ended up feeling really bad about this. Elizabeth was determined to get things as good as possible and so, following the advice of Julia, her diabetes specialist nurse, decided to try going for a walk around the block every evening after dinner. Remarkably, this did the job. The 20-minute walk round the estate and back helped to burn up a bit more of the glucose and kept her nicely in the target zone on her post-meal check – and the washing up was usually done by the time she got back!

Does exercise make much of a difference?

Yes! In addition to eating in a new way, women with diabetes in pregnancy are encouraged to exercise regularly; for example, something as simple as taking a walk for at least a half hour every day.

Even on the days when your hips hurt or your ankles are swollen, walking is a useful way to burn up the excess glucose in the system. It is straightforward and effective. Walks can be useful if your blood sugar is high, or if you know that you ate too much, then exercise can be used as a pre-emptive strike. Exercising works because muscles need extra fuel when they're active. With moderate exercise our muscles take up glucose at almost 20 times the normal resting rate. This then helps to lower blood glucose levels quickly.

What else can exercise do?

Not only can regular daily exercise during pregnancy really help with the blood glucose readings, it has several other health benefits too.

These include better fitness for the demands of labour, giving birth and breastfeeding. It also contributes to better sleep quality, helps to improve your mood and will aid with getting you back to fitness sooner after having baby. It will also give you some dedicated time for yourself during a busy day.

Any type of regular physical activity will help during pregnancy. Getting into the exercise habit is perhaps the key so that whatever you do becomes part of your routine – even a little bit every day will help.

I don't know where to begin

It's a good idea to start exercising as soon as you can in the earlier weeks of pregnancy. This will help make physical activity part of your routine. The type and the amount of exercise will evolve during the course of the pregnancy. In the first trimester you may be far too fatigued to think about doing much more than walking to the shops and back (rather than driving). In the second trimester, it's normal to get your energy back so more can be done in terms of longer, more intense walks, swimming, yoga and Pilates. In the third trimester you'll be bigger and bulkier and you may have cut back on the intensity.

How do I stay motivated? I am knackered!

It can be a good idea to exercise with a friend or another pregnant woman where possible. This can prompt you to get out of bed in the morning or get out of the house when you know someone else is waiting for you. Another method is to pay for it (gym membership or a subscription to a class). If you know that you will lose your money if you don't go, this can be enough of an incentive to get you working out.

In addition, you can plan ahead and keep your swimming things or a set of exercise clothes and sport shoes in the car or at work so you can exercise when the opportunity arises.

- Set yourself targets – these may be daily, weekly or monthly targets and could include time spent on the gym machines, distance walked, number of lengths swum – and try and improve on them slightly over time.
- Start an exercise diary. This is useful to measure your progress and record the achievements. There are also lots of smartphone apps and online charts available. In addition, there are now lots of good wearable fitness trackers on the market.
- Make a list of fun activities. Find something that you enjoy, as you'll be far more likely to keep it up. Try taking up a particular activity that the whole family or your friends can enjoy, such as swimming.
- When you are out and about it's always smart to use the stairs instead of an escalator or lift.
- Walk short journeys rather than getting in your car or taking the bus.
- To and from work, you could get off one stop early from either the bus or train.
- Use your lunch break to go for a brisk walk, or leave for any journey half an hour early in order to build in some bonus exercise time.
- If your job involves you sitting down for long periods of time, make sure that you get up regularly and walk about at intervals.

What are the safe exercise options during pregnancy?

All pregnancies are different and what you'll be able to manage can vary, sometimes from day to day or month to month. It is not uncommon for women to be affected by extreme fatigue, constant nausea, difficulty sleeping, back pains, pelvis pains and joint pains, chronic indigestion and lots of other problems. The amount and type of exercise that you'll be able to manage will be affected by all of these factors.

Simple stretches Doing 5 to 10 minutes of simple stretches once or twice per day will help to keep you supple and make a difference. This might include lower back stretches, hamstring stretches and hip opening exercises. Make sure that you don't stretch too far!

Walking This is free and easy to do and you can adjust the duration and intensity depending on your goals and energy levels.

Swimming or water aerobics This is really good non-weight bearing exercise and avoids damaging your joints.

Antenatal exercise classes Find out if there are any dedicated pregnancy classes in your local area. Such classes are good for motivation as they are done in a group. There are several antenatal yoga classes now available which are great for gentle exercise and often partners are able to join in too.

Cycling This can sometimes be slightly tricky during pregnancy as your centre of gravity and balance can change. A stationary exercise bike may be the best, and be careful to watch for pelvic pain as continued pressure from the saddle can make this worse.

Resistance work There are simple forms of resistance training in pregnancy which can be effective and easy to perform. This is useful preparation for motherhood when you will be lifting, holding and carrying baby on a regular basis. Examples of resistance exercises include sets of squats from a standing position and getting up and down from a low chair.

What should I avoid?

It's not a good idea to start an intensive or vigorous exercise programme during pregnancy. Gentle and steady are the most important things to remember. The following are not advisable when pregnant:

- intensive jogging or running
- contact sports, such as boxing or basketball
- diving
- horse riding
- trampolining
- high-intensity aerobics
- parachuting.

What about doing too much exercise and having a hypo?

If you happen to be using insulin or glibenclamide to control your blood glucose values, then you need to remember that you are at a slightly increased risk of having a hypoglycaemic episode. A hypo is not a nice experience and generally occurs when the blood glucose level gets down into the 3s. Symptoms are tiredness, irritability, confusion, hunger and sweats. Sometimes it can be difficult to recognize these symptoms if you are concentrating on the exercise so it's important to check your blood sugar levels regularly during exercise. Exercise can make you more sensitive to the action of insulin so it may be worth reducing your insulin dose slightly before exercise. The diabetes team can help guide you with this.

If you are taking insulin injections then consider these simple steps to avoiding hypoglycaemia.

- Don't inject into your muscles.
- Test your blood sugar half an hour before exercise. If it is low then it may be worth eating a small carbohydrate snack to avoid a hypoglycaemic episode following exercise.
- Test your glucose level after a period of exercise and at any point during activity if you feel unwell.
- Don't overdo it. Try to stick with mild to moderate intensity exercise.
- Always carry some carbohydrate-containing drink, food or snack with you just in case.

Anything else?

If you are able to do some regular activity that gets you up and about, then this will be really helpful in the context not only of gestational diabetes but also for your labour, your future fitness and reducing the long-term type 2 diabetes risk. Top advice for staying well includes:

- Make sure that you look after your feet – get some supportive, sensible footwear.

- Keep hydrated. Drink plenty of fluids both during and after exercise.
- Stop if it hurts. Muscle soreness and aching is normal during exercise but the onset of sudden pain isn't and it's important to ensure that you avoid injuring yourself.

6

Medication to help protect you and your baby

By week 33, Elizabeth had learnt a lot about herself, how her body reacted to certain foods, and had managed to stabilize her diabetes and get on top of the erratic blood sugar readings. Jon had helped with shopping and the cooking for their new diet, and they were both eating better overall and there was less craving for sweet foods. They were even able to spend some quality time together out of the house by going for a walk in the evenings after the main meal of the day, down to the seaside and back.

In the week leading up to her next antenatal clinic, Elizabeth had noticed that the glucose levels following her breakfast had started to rise again. The rest of the day things were okay, but it was consistently the case that she was getting readings of 7.9, 8.4 and even 9.0 on one occasion. She changed her breakfast cereal again and cut down on the portion sizes. One day she even went without any food but that just made the situation worse. She got very anxious, and when she saw Julia the diabetes specialist nurse in out-patients, she became really upset when Julia suggested that a small dose of medication would be useful at this time of day to get the blood sugar levels under control. Elizabeth burst into tears and felt like an immense failure. She had tried so hard during the second trimester to get everything right – but was now really frustrated that she would have to start metformin.

Elizabeth was not really a tablet-taking person, having never been ill in her life before. The first time she took the big white metformin tablet it felt like she was swallowing a horse pill and it made her feel really queasy for the rest of the day. After a few days however she noticed that the nausea sensation had settled down and amazingly the blood sugars after breakfast were back down, in fact better than they had been before. Elizabeth stuck with the metformin and it sorted out the problem. A few weeks later when the sugars started to rise after her evening meal, she knew that she would probably need to take some metformin with her dinner as well.

What if the diabetes gets worse despite the diet?

As the pregnancy progresses, the demands on your body get more, not less difficult to contend with. After all you are growing another human being inside you. This is hard work. The underlying disease process of **insulin resistance** can slowly get worse over the course of the pregnancy and the ability of your body to handle carbohydrates effectively lessens.

This means that, despite your dietary and lifestyle changes, the blood sugar levels can continue to go up. In some women blood sugar levels may never reach a significant stage and dietary control can be continued as the sole treatment throughout the remainder of the pregnancy; however, in others, their metabolism simply can't regulate the glucose levels enough to keep them stable.

This is very frustrating, especially if you have gone to the trouble of making major changes in the way that you prepare and eat food. Such changes will certainly have helped to reduce the glucose burden but unfortunately may not be enough on their own to do the job. It's important not to feel a failure when this happens – this is the nature of GDM, not a reflection on you.

Why are blood glucose levels often very high first thing in the morning?

One of the interesting things about regular blood glucose monitoring and the simple act of recording the results in a diary and reflecting on them is that soon patterns start to emerge. The effects of certain types of food, or different patterns of exercise, can clearly be seen and through trial and error you can begin to see what works (and more importantly what doesn't). One classic pattern that occurs with GDM is particularly difficult-to-manage blood glucose levels in the morning and after breakfast. This may take place in the absence of any other problems, with the blood glucose levels being completely fine for the rest of the day. Why does this occur? Many people might assume that it was due to a big evening meal the night before, but it's actually due to the body's normal hormonal rhythms at this particular time of day. Rises in a hormone called cortisol, for example, are usually greatest first thing in the morning and as part of its effect it can reduce the effectiveness of insulin action and lead to higher blood glucose levels. In the non-diabetic state, the body would be able to respond to this change quite quickly by simply producing more of its own insulin, but in GDM this doesn't always occur as effectively – this is generally termed insulin resistance and you may hear about this concept in several circumstances. Insulin resistance also relates to how your liver handles and stores glucose. The liver is primed to release small amounts of glucose into the bloodstream when you are between meals (overnight being generally the longest period of fasting) but in GDM, the liver can generate more glucose than usual and dump it into your system overnight.

This situation therefore creates a problem. Unlike the rises in blood sugar relating to meals and snacks which can mostly be dealt with by exercise and diet changes, this rise in morning glucose (if persistent) needs to be treated with medication to achieve good control.

Troubleshooting

High readings are frustrating. Make sure that you are getting accurate scores.

- Did you wait long enough after eating to check your CBG?
- Did you clean your hands?
- Is the glucose meter working properly? You can check this with the DSN.
- Have you missed any physical activity?
- Are you unwell or do you have a cough, a cold or a fever?
- Are you under stress or particularly emotional?

Can I try the diet for a bit longer?

This is a discussion that you need to have with your diabetes team. Hopefully, by this stage of pregnancy you should have more of a feel for the pattern of your blood glucose levels and understand the trends throughout the day. The simple act of writing down the glucose values in your booklet or diary acts as a form of feedback and reflection and often people find this far more useful than simply looking at a long string of numbers in the memory of a handheld glucose meter.

If there is an overall tendency for the blood sugars to be elevated at a particular time of day, following a particular meal or related to a specific activity, the majority of the time (i.e. more than 50 per cent of values are out of the target range), then it is worth thinking about ways in which further diet and lifestyle modifications can be made. The glucose levels can then be reassessed to see if this has worked. It may be sensible to agree on a set time frame to see if the focused changes have had an effect. It's reasonable not to leave this for too long. Our natural tendency may often be to procrastinate, see if the problem goes away by itself or ignore it, but unfortunately in pregnancy we don't have much time to play with and it's key not to spend too much time with excess glucose exposure and miss out on the right care.

The take-home message is therefore – it depends: the factors are you and your glucose levels, how out of balance the sugar values are, consideration of whether more dietary changes are likely to have an effect, and the underlying situation with your baby and how its growth and development are getting along as shown by the series of growth scans. Simply not liking the idea of going on to medication should arguably be challenged, as once treatment is started one would hope that things are not being left too late. Frequently, people comment on how much better they feel when the sugar levels are better controlled and that actually taking the medication itself is of minimal bother.

As always, talk with your team. This is about getting the situation right for you, so take advantage of their experience.

Why tablets?

When the diet changes aren't enough on their own to control blood glucose readings, the appropriate next step is to go for drug therapy to help get the sugar levels down. In the past, medical therapy largely consisted of using insulin straight away but more recently it has been found that tablet treatments can be equally good. Oral medications are an attractive alternative to insulin injections for the ease of taking them, the lower cost, and generally better acceptance. The two most commonly used tablet medications are metformin and glibenclamide. The way they work is to help improve the way in which your body handles glucose and overcome the problem of insulin resistance which is the hallmark of GDM. They work well in combination with the dietary and lifestyle changes so it's important to keep these up.

Metformin is derived from French lilac (goat's rue or *Galega officinalis*) and was used as a herbal remedy for centuries to relieve the frequent urination associated with the disease that came to be known as **diabetes mellitus** (the 'pissing evil'). It acts on the liver to improve the way in which it deals with glucose and blocks some of the liver's own glucose production – it's felt that its mechanism of action generally reduces the phenomenon of insulin resistance. Metformin is safe and effective in pregnant women and those women with GDM who use metformin have less gain in weight during pregnancy when compared to those treated with insulin. Interestingly, babies born to mothers who have used metformin develop less fat around their internal organs, and this will make them less likely to go on to develop insulin resistance and type 2 diabetes later in life.

Glibenclamide is a type of drug called a sulphonylurea and this helps to overcome the insulin issue by a different route. It acts directly on the tiny islet cells in the pancreas and stimulates them to release greater amounts of insulin. It also reduces the liver's manufacture of glucose from its own stores.

Both of these medications are best taken with meals in order to help your metabolism work more efficiently.

Is it safe to take the tablets?

One major worry of many pregnant women with GDM is whether taking any medication is safe, not only for themselves but also for their baby. This is a very reasonable question. Many modern medicines are deemed unsafe or are 'unlicensed' for use during pregnancy because they may have effects on baby's growth and development or run the risk of creating serious harm.

Fortunately, to answer this important question, there have already been several major clinical trials of pregnant women with diabetes who have used metformin and assessments have been done to look at how these large groups of individuals have got on. The results from such studies provide good evidence of the medicines' safety and show how effective they are in reducing the complications associated with GDM. Both metformin and glibenclamide are used routinely in diabetes antenatal clinics in the UK and they are good drugs in that they do what we need them to do. Rather than force any tablets on you, hopefully your diabetes team will take time to discuss and explain the potential benefits from improving your blood sugar control, as opposed to any possibility of harm. In the UK, NICE support the use of these drugs and advise that they are safe and effective for use during pregnancy.

How will it affect the baby?

The goal of the medication is to reduce the amount of time that the level of glucose in the bloodstream is outside the normal range. The risks of congenital malformations and other diabetes-associated pregnancy problems are decreased because there is a reduction in overall glucose exposure over the duration of the pregnancy; also, because of greater stability in the levels of glucose (i.e. less variation or glycaemic 'excursions'), there is less toxic harm.

Metformin has been found to be associated with fewer growth-restricted babies and a lower incidence of very low blood sugar readings in newborn babies requiring the use of a glucose infusion soon after birth. There has been no evidence of any increase in birth defects or complications at birth.

What happens if I get side effects from the medication?

The tablets for helping control blood sugar levels in GDM are good and work well in the majority of cases. However, like lots of medicines they can have side effects and it's important that you know what they potentially could be, although they do not affect everyone. If you are unlucky and do have a bad reaction, it's also useful to know whether the problems continue whenever you take the medication, or get better over time as your body gets used to the treatment. It's also difficult to say whether feeling anxious about starting a new medication in pregnancy will make you more aware of the symptoms to look out for. We usually tell people to stick with the medication for a bit to see if things get better – clearly this will be a moveable feast depending on how significant the side effects are and how much you are prepared to put up with them. If things do become intolerable, then fair enough, not all medication suits everyone and the tablets can be stopped – however, if this is the case, it's a good idea to get directly in contact with your diabetes team so that the next steps can be talked about, rather than wait two weeks until your next appointment and continue to have high glucose levels.

Common side effects of metformin

One of the most frequently reported side effects is gastro-intestinal upset. This covers a multitude of problems with your tummy and bowels – anything from feeling bloated and gassy, a funny metallic feeling in the mouth, feeling sick and more likely to vomit, to more exaggerated symptoms like diarrhoea, stomach cramps and bowel spasms. Some people can have very dramatic reactions and don't want to take it again while others get just a mild tummy upset, or loss of appetite, which settles down after a few days. These side effects are usually less bad if metformin is taken with a meal. Metformin can also cause skin reactions and occasionally low blood sugars. Metformin should be used with caution in people with kidney, heart and liver problems; usually your clinicians will be aware if these are relevant problems for you and avoid using it.

Common side effects of glibenclamide

The biggest problem to watch for with any of the sulphonylurea class of medications is that of hypoglycaemia – they are very good at doing what they are supposed to (stimulating insulin production) and dropping your blood sugar levels. Rarely, glibenclamide can also cause tummy upset, skin reactions and headaches. Glibenclamide shouldn't be used if you have a condition called **G6PD deficiency** as it may cause a reaction with your red blood cells.

I don't want to take any tablets

Nobody will pressure you to take any medication that you are uncomfortable with taking. Consider it as a menu of options being presented to you. The best thing is to be well informed about why the medications are being suggested, what they are likely to do and their risks and benefits. This then allows you to make the best choices for you and baby. You should always have the option of being able to go away, have a think, come back and talk things through in as much detail as you want – even in a busy clinic setting where you may feel in a rush. Pregnancy can be a difficult time and going onto medication may go against ideas of a natural pregnancy or relate to a general dislike of the concept of taking tablets.

Most pregnant women with GDM follow the standard treatment plan, so give the medications a try and see how you get on with them and if they do the job of getting the glucose levels under control. If it seems like your antenatal team are rather insistent that going onto medication is the best thing for you, then it's usually because they wouldn't want you missing out on the best treatments. Hopefully, you will feel comfortable discussing your concerns with them in an open manner – but admittedly this isn't always easy.

What happens if the tablets don't work?

The main problem with oral medicines used for diabetes (apart from their potential side effects described above) is that they may not work for everyone with GDM. Generally, you should start to see an improvement in the blood sugar levels after meals within a few days and if you are recording the values in a record book it's nice to see how the pattern changes. However, if there is no improvement, the next step is for the dose of the drug to be increased. For example, most people will start on 500 milligrams of metformin with breakfast and dinner. If the dose needs upping to get on top of the glucose levels, then the dose may be changed to either 850 milligrams three times per day (with each of the main meals) or 1000 milligrams with breakfast and dinner instead – it depends on how you respond.

If you are stepped up to the top dose of metformin (or gliben-clamide) and are taking it regularly for a decent period of time and tolerating it okay, then it should be clear whether it has worked or not – are the majority of the finger prick glucose readings now in the target range?

If not, then it may be that the GDM is more advanced and despite the medication, your body is unable to get those glucose levels down to where you need them to be. If this is the case then it is clear that there is still a large element of insulin resistance – this important hormone is not being produced in sufficient amounts to control your metabolism. The time has therefore come to give you additional insulin.

What does insulin do?

Insulin is the key hormone which controls glucose levels in the bloodstream. It's a messenger which allows glucose to get from the circulation into the tissues and into the brain and get to work. As described before, GDM is an insulin-resistant state, meaning that your own insulin production simply doesn't work as well as it should and we need to get extra insulin into you to compensate for this.

How is insulin given?

Insulin has to be given as an injection into the fatty layer under the skin (subcutaneously) as it can't be absorbed from the gut in

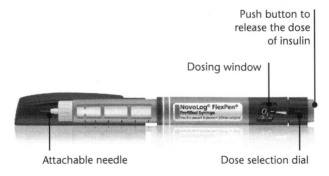

Push button to release the dose of insulin

Dosing window

Attachable needle   Dose selection dial

Figure 6.1 Insulin pen

the same way that tablets are. Insulin normally comes in a pen-like device with a cartridge containing the hormone and can be fitted with a very small needle for doing the injection (Figure 6.1 on the previous page). There is often a lot of trepidation and anxiety over injecting insulin. This is often disproportionate to the realities of doing the injection, which many people find far more straightforward and less painful than doing the finger prick glucose check.

If you need to take insulin, you will be shown how and where to inject yourself, normally in an easily accessible, fleshy part of your body, such as your stomach (round the sides, away from baby), thighs or upper arms – even the top of the buttocks can be used. In addition, you'll need to know how to store your insulin (usually in the fridge before it is first used – it's fine out of the fridge for a month) and how to get rid of the disposable needles (you should be provided with a bright yellow sharps bin). The diabetes team will also tell you about recognizing the signs and symptoms of low blood glucose (and how to treat this by yourself), and finally you should be given the updated information about driving and the DVLA regulations with regard to insulin – given that it is only a temporary treatment the rules are not that strict. More information can be found at <www.gov.uk/guidance/assessing-fitness-to-drive-a-guide-for-medical-professionals>.

Generally the guidance is that you should notify the DVLA if treatment continues for more than 3 months in the context of GDM.

What are the different types of insulin?

Insulin comes in several different types and preparations. They can also have confusingly similar names, so you need to make sure that your GP gets your repeat prescription correct. The broad categories of insulin relate to how long they last in the body. 'Quick acting' or 'short acting' insulin, for example, is usually given with meals to counter the surge in glucose entering the bloodstream. It gets to work within 15 minutes or so and its effects generally last for 2 to 4 hours. In contrast, there are 'long acting' insulins which are designed to keep the background levels of glucose under control; these normally start to exert an effect an hour or so after injection

Table 6.1 Classes of insulin

Class of insulin	Examples	Time-action profile
Short / quick acting	Insulin aspart (Novo-Rapid), insulin glulisine (Apidra), insulin lispro (Humalog)	Gets to work within 30 minutes and is generally out of the system over the next 2 to 4 hours
Intermediate acting	Isophane insulins (Insulatard, Humulin I)	Onset is within 2 hours, has a peak effect around 4 hours and then starts to slowly fade away over about 16–18 hours
Long acting	Insulin glargine (Lantus), insulin detemir (Levemir)	Rises to a plateau concentration in the blood within 1 to 2 hours and then stays at relatively stable levels for 20–24 hours

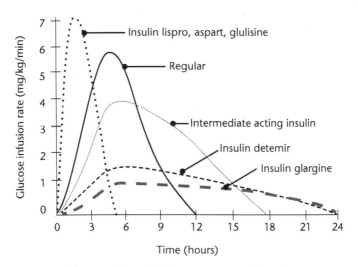

Figure 6.2 Activity profiles of different types of insulin

and can last much longer, i.e. over 20 hours – this means that you may only need to take them once or twice per day (Table 6.1 and Figure 6.2 on the previous page).

Establishing the right combination of different insulins needs to be tailored to you. It may be that you only require a small dose of quick acting insulin with your breakfast and nothing else. It could alternatively be that the pre-meal values are high across the board, so you need to be treated with a long acting insulin once in the morning and once in the evening. There are several different approaches to getting insulin into you and these relate to the pattern of your capillary blood glucose (**CBG**) monitoring, which will help determine your combination.

How do I give myself an insulin injection?

When this medication is prescribed it is standard practice to talk through the kit with you and show you how it's used. Don't panic, it's all actually rather straightforward. The needles on the insulin pen are very small and the places where you give the injection have a lot fewer sensory nerve fibres (as compared to your fingertips, which are some of the most sensitive parts of your whole body).

First of all:

- Take off the cap of the insulin pen device and screw on a new needle for each injection.
- Pull back the button on the end and twist to dial up 2 units (a number 2 should appear in the small window).
- Then push the plunger down so that a small amount of liquid comes out the tip of the needle. This is to prime the needle and remove any air.

Now you're ready to go:

- Dial up the required dose.
- Pick a soft fatty area to inject (the best places are the sides of your abdomen or tummy area, upper outer arms, thighs or the top of the buttocks) and take a pinch of fatty flesh between your thumb and forefinger – making sure that there is space in between.
- Then put the needle straight in. A 90-degree angle is normally

fine; however, you can go at 45 degrees if you are particularly slim – this is in order to avoid injecting too deeply down into muscle.

- Slowly push the plunger down to inject the dose.
- Hold the needle in place and slowly count to 10 – this prevents too much insulin escaping.
- Withdraw and then unscrew the needle and dispose into a sharps bin.

What are the side effects of insulin?

Insulin is safe in pregnancy, but it is important that you check your blood glucose levels on a regular basis, as there is a risk of hypoglycaemia – more on this below. One of the other effects of insulin is that it is an anabolic-type hormone and this can predispose to some weight gain when taken in excess. It is important therefore to monitor your sugar levels and work with your diabetes team to make sure that the doses of insulin that you are on are ideally adjusted to suit you. Weight gain may be related to the more efficient use of calories, which suggests that there will be extra benefits of exercise and dietary changes. Patients on an 'intensive' insulin therapy regime (4 or 5 injections per day) may be more likely to have problems with weight gain.

Other side effects may relate to irritation or stinging at the site of an injection. You can get a fatty reaction in the tissues under the skin if you keep injecting in the same place for a long time; this is called lipodystrophy and is best avoided by making sure that you regularly change whereabouts on your body you inject your insulin. With any treatment that breaks the skin there is also the risk of infection if the site is not clean. It is also important to change the needles for every injection.

I am scared of needles!

This is not an unreasonable thing to think in the situation where you have gone from being a completely healthy individual, to suddenly being told that you have to give yourself one or more injections per day and that this may involve some discomfort.

Unfortunately, we can't get insulin into you in any other way, so it has to be given through the skin into the fatty tissue below the surface. If you have already been doing the finger prick check on a daily basis then it's good to know that an actual insulin injection is much less painful. The nerves in the fingertips are far more concentrated and sensitive to being stabbed than the places where the insulin is supposed to go. Also the needles used with modern insulin injection devices are much finer and smaller than the historic vials and syringes that were once used.

Going on to insulin can be a very big deal for some people and needle phobia can play a part in this. You are not alone. One simple way round it is to do a dummy injection with your diabetes practitioner in the antenatal clinic. People's commonest reaction to this is 'Is that it?' or 'What was all the fuss about?' If you are anxious then it's important to talk to other mums in the clinic and to your diabetes team about your worries – they will have seen lots of people with the same issue and have ways of coping. Nobody wants you to miss out on the best treatment.

My diabetes team keep telling me to write down the CBG readings in a book or a diary – why can't they just look at them in the meter memory?

One of the major ways in which we help to manage diabetes is using the patterns of blood glucose values to work out what is going on. There is a fair amount of research which has shown that those people who actively write down their readings, review the results and reflect on the changes required, tend to do much better in both the short and the long term. It's a good habit to get into as it means that you pay more attention to your diabetes, and if you look at the format in which most blood glucose data is represented then it can make it easier for you and your healthcare team to identify where the pinch points are, what are the problematic times of day and which of the medications may need to be adjusted to help solve the issue. This is nowhere near as easy when looking through a context-free string of numbers on the screen of a glucose meter (which often don't have the right date and time settings anyway).

Table 6.2 Glucose readings

	Before breakfast	1 hour after breakfast	Before lunch	1 hour after lunch	Before dinner	1 hour after dinner	Before bedtime
Monday	4.5	6.9	4.9	6.6		8.4	
Tuesday	5.1	7.9			4.6	9.2	4.7
Wednesday			5.0	7.1	4.5	8.7	
Thursday	3.8	8.0	3.9	5.8	5.0	7.9	
Friday	4.4	8.5	4.1	6.2	6.3	9.1	5.9
Saturday	4.8				4.4	10.2	9.2
Sunday		8.8	3.7	5.9	3.9	7.7	

Table 6.2 demonstrates the point about context. In this example it is clear that the glucose values are running high after meals (while it's not happening all the time, it is forming a trend) and more than half of the values are out of target after breakfast and the evening meal. This suggests that the background (or fasting) blood glucose control is okay, but when a meal is taken, there is an uncontrolled rise in the glucose values. This would be an indication under the circumstances for starting metformin with those two meals. If already on metformin, it's clear that more is needed and the dose

Table 6.3 Second set of glucose readings

	Before breakfast	1 hour after breakfast	Before lunch	1 hour after lunch	Before dinner	1 hour after dinner	Before bedtime
Monday	12.2	16.2	13.0		11.3		
Tuesday	13.1	15.0	11.9	9.4		15.1	16.0
Wednesday	9.2	11.1	8.6	7.7	10.2	13.2	9.8
Thursday	8.7	9.9		10.3		12.3	10.2
Friday	6.9	8.4	8.9	7.8	9.4	10.5	12.3
Saturday	9.8		10.3	12.2	13.1		
Sunday	8.5	10.2			9.6	13.2	

can be increased, generally to a maximum dose of 1 gram twice a day or 850 milligrams three times a day. If we are already on the top dose of metformin then we've got to a state of significant insulin resistance and we need to go onto some quick acting insulin doses with meals in addition to the insulin. The dose of this can then be adjusted according to the subsequent post-meal checks – often only a very small dose is required.

Table 6.3 has a second set of readings that demonstrate high blood glucose values both before and after meals. It would make sense to think therefore that the background glucose levels are uncontrolled and running high; rather than dealing with the higher post-meal values as before, now is the time to do something about the high before-meal readings (the fasting hyperglycaemia). The first course of action is to adopt the lifestyle and dietary measures previously discussed in Chapters 3, 4 and 5. If these do not succeed then the best way of treating persistent fasting hyperglycaemia is to introduce a once-a-day shot of long acting insulin such as Lantus (insulin glargine), which is given as an injection once per day and acts in a slow release manner to keep the background blood sugars under control (a general dampener). This treatment helps to bring those higher before-meal values down and consequently the ones after the meals will not be as elevated; indeed it may be a good way of getting them back into the target range and avoiding extra treatment.

The principles outlined above are used to guide the adjustment of tablet and insulin therapy throughout pregnancy. Sometimes it is hard to identify a pattern, so cautious changes will be made. The diabetes team will be experienced in analysing glucose profiles and making suggestions to help guide the tweaking of blood glucose lowering therapies. One thing that is always nice to see in clinic is when a woman with GDM gets more comfortable and confident with reviewing her own blood glucose values and making cautious adjustments to her own treatment. So long as you are happy to do this it should be perfectly acceptable to make sensible changes yourself – but don't worry if you're not!

What should I do if I have a hypo?

As soon as you realize that you are having a hypoglycaemic episode – either because you have taken a capillary blood glucose reading or are starting to get signs and symptoms of a low sugar level – then it needs treating straightaway. It's not something that can be left to sort itself out. If treatment is delayed you might start to get drowsy or forget what you are doing. The worst case scenario is that you pass out completely. Rarely, people can have a seizure with a severe hypo.

The signs and symptoms of a hypo are: feeling light-headed, dizzy, sweaty, confused, irritable and/or hungry, drowsiness, weakness and shakes.

The right treatment for a hypo is to get the blood sugar back up to normal as speedily as possible by taking carbohydrates. It can be brought up within minutes by taking the right type of food or drink. For example: 50–100 ml of unsweetened fruit juice or Lucozade; 4–5 dextrose tablets or 4–5 jelly babies are also good. It's a sensible idea to always carry some hypo treatment with you and make it easily accessible for when you are out and about so it can be used quickly if need be. Avoid chocolate as this is fatty and is slower to be absorbed. Eating lots and lots of carbohydrate (overfeeding) at this stage doesn't really help and doesn't speed recovery (although you may feel desperately hungry) and runs the risk of subsequent hyperglycaemia.

After you've taken some treatment, it's a good idea to recheck the glucose level after 15 minutes or so to make sure that things are improving. If it's still low at that stage then it's a good idea to take some longer acting carbohydrate to help keep the blood sugars up and stop the hypo from happening again.

If you become so drowsy and unwell that you can't manage to eat or drink anything yourself to help the hypo, then this is a more serious situation. Make sure that your partner, friends, family and work colleagues are aware that you are prone to hypoglycaemia and know how to help treat this, or at least call for help. It may be necessary to get a paramedic to attend to give a sugary substance called Hypostop and glucose containing fluid intravenously or to inject you with a medication called glucagon, which helps to quickly bring up the blood sugar levels.

What can I do to stop a hypo from happening in the first place?

It's important to prevent hypos from happening in the first place and to try and identify why they have occurred when they do. A common cause of hypoglycaemia is not eating enough food in relation to the dose of insulin that has been injected – a mismatch that can be discussed with your diabetes dietician. Other factors include exercise, stress, alcohol, stimulants such as caffeine, exertion, or delay in eating, e.g. slow delivery of food in a restaurant – don't inject until your food arrives!

If you are suffering from frequent or severe hypoglycaemia then it is important to reduce the offending insulin doses and pay close attention to glucose levels, perhaps by more frequent monitoring. More regular low GI snacking may be an alternative way around the problem. Some quick acting insulins may bring down your glucose to a satisfactory level one hour after the meal, but then continue to act and drop the glucose level further and make you at risk of hypoglycaemia a few hours after eating.

What should I do if I have a very high blood glucose reading?

The answer to this question really depends on the timing and the circumstances. Multiple interfering factors can cause a high reading, as can poor injection technique and missing or forgetting the insulin. Symptoms of high blood glucose include feeling tired and irritable, passing lots of urine, being very thirsty and blurring of your eyesight.

If your glucose level is high before a meal it may be that you need to give yourself a corrective dose (an additional amount) alongside the regular mealtime insulin dose in order to get the blood sugar level back to normal.

If the sugar levels are consistently high at this time then it is likely that you need more of the long acting background insulin in your system on a regular basis.

If the glucose is high at random times between meals it may be necessary to give yourself an extra shot of insulin to get things back to normal, especially if you are up in the high teens or 20s. Make sure that this is a true reading however, as having unclean hands with food residue on them can give a false reading (you should speak with your diabetes team about how much extra quick acting insulin to give at such times as everyone will be slightly different).

What happens if I don't want to inject myself with insulin?

In the context of GDM it is likely that the blood glucose levels will continue to be high and this will then lead on to the increased risks associated with diabetes in pregnancy: large babies, malformations and higher risks of miscarriage and stillbirth, etc. It is of course by no means definite that these things will happen, but it certainly puts you into the high-risk pregnancy category. Some clinicians may attempt to scare you with stories of what can go wrong and make you feel guilty for not being a 'compliant' patient, but so long as you are well informed and understand the risks and can discuss these in a blame-free environment then nobody can make you go on to insulin (or do anything else you don't want to, for that matter).

Will I have to stay on insulin for life?

No. For the vast majority of people with GDM, the condition goes away as soon as baby is born. It is as quick as that. Your metabolism reverts to normal, the insulin resistant state melts away and you don't need the insulin any more. You may only end up taking insulin for a few weeks or a few months depending at which stage of pregnancy you need to go onto it.

There are of course some individuals who may have ongoing diabetes (either type 1 or type 2) that is uncovered during pregnancy, but is usually possible to identify these individuals and keep them under review.

I am very busy – I'm not used to taking medication every day. What can I do?

Remembering when to take your medications can be tricky, especially with the many pressures in life, and it can be a challenge to look after yourself and fit everything into your daily routine. There are a few ways round this:

- Get into the habit – organize taking any medication into your regular routine. Have the tablets next to where you make the morning coffee or use sticky notes in a prominent position to catch your eye to remind you. You can even set a reminder alarm on your phone.
- Weekly pill sorter or 'dosette' box. Your GP can arrange for your local pharmacy to put all your tablets into a container with clear date and time reminders to let you keep track of what you have taken.
- Keep standbys and spares. It's always important to keep your insulin kit and your glucose meter with you when out and about. It may be worth keeping a spare insulin pen in your bag or in the car so that you've always got something close at hand and won't miss a dose.
- Smartphone apps – there are several apps out there, which help track and remind you to take your medication.

Why is it sometimes difficult to get my blood glucose levels under control?

Ever-changing levels of glucose can be par for the course with GDM. It is not unusual to find that blood sugar levels appear to go up and down with no clear explanation.

It is useful to remember that it is not just the effects of eating food which can cause the glucose to fluctuate. Other factors include stress, emotion, activity and exercise, alcohol, the time of day (the morning, for example, can be a time of significantly greater insulin resistance), or the day of the week (having a lie in or getting up later on a weekend can prolong the fasting time and cause your liver to start making glucose of its own).

Other causes of blood glucose swings are:

- *Sugar free or 'low sugar' foods* are products which still have carbohydrates in them in the form of starches and sugar alcohols (for example, fructose or sorbitol). These additives give food flavour and make things taste sweet but can still disturb your glucose levels.
- *Caffeine* has a stimulant effect, so even without any extra added calories from milk or sugar, a cup of tea or coffee can cause a rise in the blood sugar.
- *Medications* Tablets taken to treat other medical conditions can impact on the blood sugar control. Make sure you find out whether this is included in their list of side effects. Steroids such as hydrocortisone and prednisolone can make diabetes worse; other drugs such as frusemide or bendrofluazide (diuretics used for fluid retention) and several anti-depressants (such as Citalopram) can interfere. However don't stop taking them until you have spoken to your healthcare team.
- *High-fat foods* can make your glucose levels stay higher for longer; lots of fat plus lots of carbs doesn't work well. Examples include chips, pizza and takeaways.
- *Stress* Problems at home, in your relationships or at work can affect your body and cause the release of certain stress hormones. Try to take stock of what may be upsetting you and think about various relaxation options such as meditation, exercise, yoga and deep breathing.
- *Heat* Higher temperatures make blood sugar control more difficult and can also predispose you to dehydration. If you are heavily pregnant during a hot summer then make sure that you drink lots of fluid and check your glucose more regularly.
- *Illness* If an infection such as a bout of flu or even the common cold occurs, your body's natural stress reaction is to push up the blood sugar levels. This can be made worse by dehydration, so make sure that you keep your fluid intake up. Some medicines such as antibiotics or cold and flu relief treatments can also interfere, e.g. pseudoephedrine.
- *Exertion* Any vigorous activity, either sustained or in short bursts (running for a bus, for example), may be enough to burn up the

glucose in your system and precipitate a drop in the blood sugar levels. While exercise is a very good way to help control glucose levels, some people can be very sensitive and have a tendency to make their blood glucose go too low. When you are active enough to raise your heart rate and break a sweat there may be a temporary surge in the glucose level, followed by a marked drop. Think about taking a snack before you begin in order to help balance things out. It's a good idea to check your capillary blood glucose levels before the exercise, during and afterwards as well.

What causes hypoglycaemia?

Many of the above factors can bring about low levels of glucose. The general factors are usually not eating enough, taking too much medication relative to what you are eating, or too much exertion. It's best to avoid this situation by eating regularly, making sure that you are not taking excessive carbohydrates out of your diet (both you and baby need the fuel), monitoring your blood sugars regularly and recording the results, and checking that you are giving your insulin medication in the right way (and not accidentally taking too much).

You are never harming yourself or doing something wrong by taking a glucose tablet or some hypo treatment if you suspect that you are having a hypo.

Do very low blood sugar readings hurt my baby?

This is a very genuine concern – the thought that a very low level of glucose can cause harm. The management of gestational diabetes can often be thought of as a tightrope – making sure that most of the time the sugars are not too high while trying to avoid swinging too far in the opposite direction and becoming hypoglycaemic can be a difficult balance.

Hypoglycaemia in the mother does not harm the unborn baby as much as hyperglycaemia, but recurrent, severe episodes can cause problems. When you have a hypo, there are mechanisms in place to protect the baby and make sure that its glucose levels are maintained. There is generally a metabolic reaction which triggers the release of glucose stores in order to continue the supply. Intermittent episodes of mild treated hypoglycaemia are very unlikely to create any significant damage to baby or its growth. Babies are generally very resilient.

Hypoglycaemia is perhaps more of a concern for the effects that it has on the pregnant mother. Lack of glucose to the brain can affect the way that you think and feel, cause agitation or drowsiness, clumsiness and poor concentration. When your brain doesn't work properly you are more at risk of having a fall or accident and harming the baby or yourself that way.

Severe, prolonged hypoglycaemia (several hours or more, rather than a few minutes) rarely occurs, but could potentially lead to brain damage if there is a long period when not enough glucose is getting to baby's brain. This would be very unusual and is unlikely to occur without some form of prior warning.

If you are having problems with lots of episodes of hypoglycaemia, or are losing awareness of becoming hypoglycaemic (which is actually very unusual in GDM), then your treatment combination or pattern of eating needs looking at and adjusting to avoid the problem happening. Speak with your midwife or diabetes team – don't wait until your next appointment. If there is a problem with achieving the target glucose values, then they may be adjusted to suit you more and avoid the hypos.

7

Progressing in later pregnancy

By the time Elizabeth had reached the third trimester, she was getting larger and more exhausted than ever. Apart from the swollen ankles, the cramps in her back and the pains in her pelvis, she still had the GDM to deal with. She'd generally been getting on well with her blood sugar control and the medications were less of a bother. One particular outing to a local restaurant for a birthday party had been a disaster with very high blood sugars for a whole day afterwards but other than that she was managing okay.

The visits every fortnight to the antenatal clinic were useful and reassuring and it was nice to be able to see the baby on the regular growth scans. She didn't always get to see the same team members but the pregnancy notes she carried round with her contained a clear plan, and everyone seemed to know what was going on (most of the time) and all the right checks and tests were being done. Elizabeth was in fact very keen to make sure that she kept herself in good health after the pregnancy to try and avoid getting diabetes in the future – she certainly didn't want to have to go through all of this in her next pregnancy (not that she was planning it just yet!). Overall, she felt that she was getting into the groove of GDM and was happier now that she knew what she was doing and why.

Why do I keep needing to have blood tests?

Throughout the pregnancy, it is important to ensure that regular checks are being done which guide your treatment. They are also useful for screening for potential complications. All the blood tests offered are being done for the health of you and your baby, not to satisfy the doctors or to annoy you.

For example, the HbA1c blood test (glycosylated haemoglobin) should be performed at regular intervals to show that the overall blood glucose control is stable and not deteriorating. Generally, it is the pattern that HbA1c comes down during pregnancy as a reflection of improvements in diet, the effects of medication and an overall reduction in glucose exposure. If the HbA1c is creeping upwards, then it suggests that it is time to tighten up the glucose control. HbA1c is traditionally measured as a percentage. A reading of 6.0 per cent or lower suggests that the average glucose control is good. Above this, the results suggest that the sugar levels have been elevated and in the diabetic range for some time. More and more centres are switching to measurement of HbA1c in units of millimoles per mole (mmol/mol). The upper limit of the non-diabetic range is 42 mmol/mol and is the equivalent of 6.0 per cent.

Other blood tests commonly performed in the antenatal diabetes clinic include liver function tests (LFTs) which tell us about the behaviour of various enzymes within the liver. One recognized complication of pregnancy which we occasionally see is called **obstetric cholestasis**, which describes an impaired flow of bile from the gall bladder (this can often be associated with a marked itchiness) and this can be picked up on the LFTs.

You may hear the term U&Es, which stands for 'urea and electrolytes'. This tells us about your kidney function, as can a particular urine test called an ACR (albumin:creatinine ratio) which shows us whether there is any leakage of small amounts of protein from the kidneys into the urine.

In addition, a full blood count (FBC) test tells us about the production of haemoglobin – the red blood cells which carry oxygen around the body. A low level of haemoglobin is called anaemia and during pregnancy this has several causes, including iron deficiency. It can be another contributing factor to making you feel tired and run down. You will also have a check of your blood group just in case you need a blood transfusion at any point.

Along with checking the total amount of haemoglobin, it's common to check pregnant women for any diseases of the red blood cells which could affect their ability to carry oxygen around the body. Haemoglobinopathy refers to disorders of these cells, which tend to run in families. Testing for such blood cell disorders can tell you whether you have this problem and whether it is likely that it will be passed on to your children.

It's also common to check you for infectious diseases which could potentially affect your pregnancy or be transferred to baby; the standard tests include Rubella or German measles immunity, HIV, Hepatitis B and Syphilis. You can also have a blood test for Hepatitis C if you are felt to be at high risk. If any of these tests are positive then your team will contact you as soon as possible and explain about effective treatments for you and baby.

What else...?

Blood pressure testing You'll get used to the fact that at most appointments the midwives or the maternity care assistants (MCAs) will check your blood pressure (BP). The results will be compared to the ones from early pregnancy to make sure that it is not on the rise. It's not unusual for your blood pressure to be on the high side when you come to clinic; this can be due to the anxiety and stimulation of coming to the hospital and is sometimes called white coat hypertension. It normally settles down on repeat testing. If your blood pressure is always on the high side or creeping up then you'll be checked out to make sure that you have no signs of **pre-eclampsia** or pregnancy-induced hypertension (high blood pressure).

Urine testing You may be asked to produce a wee sample and this can be tested using a dipstick to check for protein and glucose. Glucose in the urine, as we know, suggests diabetes and protein in the urine can be a sign of either a bladder infection, primary kidney disease or high blood pressure/pre-eclampsia.

How often can I expect an ultrasound scan?

The general pattern of surveillance scans during pregnancy are for an initial ultrasound at 12 weeks gestation (sometimes called a viability scan) to make sure that baby is okay and growing properly, that the pregnancy is viable – likely to continue. This is followed by a 20-week scan, sometimes called a mid-pregnancy or anomaly scan, which is done to look for any signs of unusual development (Figure 7.1).

In the 20-week scan, the scanner (ultrasonographer) should specifically be checking for the shape and size of baby's head, looking at baby's face for a cleft lip and palate, checking the spine, the

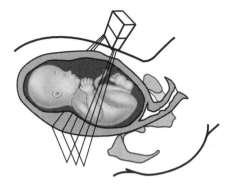

Figure 7.1 Cross-sectional image of an antenatal ultrasound scan

heart, the baby's tummy to make sure that all the internal organs are in place, the limbs, hands and feet and the placenta as well as the umbilical cord. This all involves quite a lot of measuring and checking. Don't be surprised if the scanner is really quiet while doing all these checks – it's not because there is anything wrong, it's because the scanner is really concentrating! The 20-week scan can also reveal whether you are having a boy or a girl, but the scanner won't tell you without first checking that you want to know.

The scanner purposefully checks for a set list of conditions including heart defects and spina bifida; some conditions may be difficult to see and some are very rare, but important. It's like getting a very thorough MOT. The things checked for are either very serious – which could affect baby's survival – or the scanner may pick up a treatable condition which can be tackled once baby is born. The scanner doesn't always get a good view, so he or she may ask you to come back when baby is lying in a different position.

For those without diabetes or other conditions (such as having an underactive thyroid) which need checking during pregnancy, that is all the standard scanning which takes place.

Now, with GDM, type 1 and type 2 diabetes, more scans are needed to check on how well baby is developing over the latter course of pregnancy because of the concerns about growth patterns – that is growing excessively and getting too large, or not growing well enough, sometimes called growth restriction. You

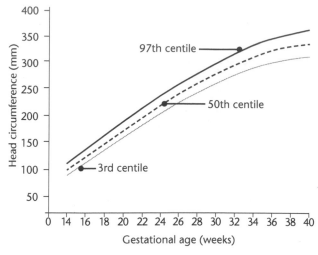

Figure 7.2 Pattern of baby head-size growth

Note Chart to show the pattern of baby head-size growth during pregnancy, based on international standards developed by the University of Oxford

may hear the term IUGR, which stands for intra-uterine growth restriction.

Growth scans will subsequently take place in a series at regular intervals throughout the remainder of your pregnancy. Serial growth scanning is a useful way of assessing the baby's growth and comparing it to average patterns of baby development. A growth chart is shown in Figure 7.2 which plots how the baby's head circumference changes over time. The measurement lines are called centiles and you may hear reference to population averages, which is a way of comparing your baby's growth to others. For example, growing along the fiftieth centile – in the middle – suggests that baby has a completely average measurement. Anything between the upper and lower lines represents a normal measurement, and the obstetricians will generally be most interested in how the measurements are changing over time in relation to the standard growth plots. The upper line is called the ninety-seventh centile and growth above this level may be a concern.

If a baby starts off on the large side and remains on the large side without veering wildly off course then this represents normal growth. However, if there are changes in the trajectory of growth over time, e.g. crossing the centiles and getting smaller or significantly bigger over time, then it will become clear on the charts. The series, rather than the absolute values, are what is most important here. One-off anomalous measurements may not mean much if the overall trend of growth is consistent (and we know that babies tend to grow at uneven rates).

Different antenatal clinics use scanning in slightly different ways. It is most common to have a growth scan every 4 weeks as this is sufficient to assess changes in growth. There is little evidence to suggest that more frequent scanning makes much of a difference. Although it is nice to see your baby on the monitor and know that baby is doing well when you come to the antenatal clinic every fortnight, don't be surprised or disappointed if you don't get a scan every time you attend. There's also no medical reason to pay for a **4D scan**, as this doesn't provide any extra information that would change what is being done in the diabetes antenatal clinic.

Finally, your midwife will also arrange for you to have a dedicated heart scan for baby if you have pre-existing diabetes. This is because of the slightly increased risk of heart problems occurring. This scan generally takes place around 18–22 weeks and may have to be done in a specialist centre in a bigger hospital elsewhere. Don't be surprised if you are asked to travel to a different hospital to get this done – it's an important scan.

How accurate are growth scans?

It may be that when you have several ultrasound scans close together, some of the measurements will seem different in a short space of time. There are several explanations for this. It could be due to different scanning technicians or obstetricians performing the measurements on different occasions; it could be due to the ultrasound machine itself and how good a view it provides. It can also depend on the position of baby and whether a good view can be obtained. Some centres no longer provide an estimated foetal weight because the measurements are known to be unreliable and concentrate on abdominal and head circumference instead.

We know that growth scan measurements can vary, so it is important that (as with blood sugars) the trend over time is looked at rather than the individual values. One interesting and useful website is <www.baby2see.com/medical/charts.html>. This website allows you to put in your own measurements and helps to calculate gestational age, due date and birth weight – but as with all these things, take the results with a pinch of salt.

What happens if baby is not growing as well as expected?

Growth restriction is more likely in smokers, women aged over 40, women who are obese, those with a poor diet, women who use cocaine, those with high blood pressure and those with a background history of previous small babies or stillbirths. Stopping smoking can stop some babies from developing intra-uterine growth restriction.

If it appears that baby is not growing as well as expected, you and the baby will require extra monitoring. It may be that the baby will need to be delivered earlier than planned. There are several risks associated with growth restriction which include miscarriage and stillbirth, low oxygen levels and distress during labour, and hypoglycaemia after being born.

The extra tests will usually involve weekly growth scans, a Doppler ultrasound to measure the blood flow through the umbilical artery and measurement of the amount of amniotic fluid (sometimes known as liquor) around the baby.

What happens if the baby gets too large?

The growth scans may show that the baby is getting too big and crossing centiles or shooting over the ninety-seventh centile on the growth chart. This is a concern. Babies weighing, or predicted to weigh, more than 4.5 kilos are considered to be larger than average (usually deemed to be about 3.1 kilos). Macrosomia, 'big body', occurs in about 5 to 10 per cent of pregnancies and GDM is probably the biggest risk factor for this happening.

A big baby leads to the possibility of more problems when giving birth; problems for baby include obstructed labour and shoulder dystocia (where the shoulder gets stuck behind the pubic bone), which can sometimes result in a broken collarbone and reduced oxygen levels to baby's brain, potentially causing permanent damage. These situations are rare but they do need immediate treatment to prevent severe injury or death. If a large baby is suspected, then it is unlikely that the obstetricians or midwives would support a home delivery. The risks to mother include pelvic trauma and perineal damage and increased bleeding following delivery.

In terms of management, from the GDM perspective, there will be increased pressure to ensure that the blood sugar control is optimal and this could necessitate further improvements in diet (not diet restriction), increasing medication doses, starting on insulin or cranking up the insulin doses.

From the obstetric point of view, your doctor will have a talk with you about the best ways to manage delivering a large baby. You may get even more frequent ultrasound scans to monitor how baby is doing and you will need to consider either induction of labour at an earlier stage of gestation (i.e. having baby before term) or a caesarean section if the risks of a normal vaginal delivery are thought to be too great.

Why do I need to be admitted to hospital for steroid treatment?

For various reasons, based on individual circumstances, baby may need to be delivered earlier than the normal 40 weeks of gestation. Clearly, the baby may not be fully mature and one of the biggest complications of earlier than normal delivery is foetal lung immaturity. This describes the situation whereby a newborn baby's lungs aren't able to do their job and help the baby to breathe adequately. Steroids also reduce the risks of bleeding within the brain and death during labour. The steroids (either dexamethasone or betamethasone) are given as a course of two injections, 12 hours apart, usually into your thigh muscle or buttocks.

One of the classic side effects of steroid treatments is that they interfere with carbohydrate metabolism and cause blood glucose levels to rise. Therefore in patients with GDM there exists the possibility of rampantly high glucose readings for 1 to 2 days following an injection of steroids. Most obstetric departments will already have a clear management plan relating to the use of steroids for mothers with diabetes in pregnancy. In some cases, it may be that nothing more than frequent monitoring is required to make sure the glucose levels come down and this may or may not require an in-patient stay on the antenatal ward. In other circumstances the glucose levels may rise so much (and not come down) that an intravenous drip with fluids and insulin is temporarily required to bring the glucose levels back under control. Usually this is a short-lived effect and things stabilize, but in some people it can take frustratingly long for things to come back to normal.

Are there other medical complications that may occur as a consequence of gestational diabetes?

GDM is also known to cause an increase in the risk of premature birth (baby being born before 37 weeks) and this can lead to problems such as respiratory distress and newborn jaundice. There is also the possibility of baby being hypoglycaemic soon after birth and needing to go to the special care baby unit (SCBU) to be given glucose. High blood glucose levels from the mother stimulate high insulin levels in the baby.

Apart from macrosomia, the other congenital malformations that GDM may cause include:

- heart disorders such as a hole in the heart and transposition of the great arteries;
- nervous system problems such as spina bifida;
- kidney problems such as underdevelopment of the kidneys;
- skeletal problems, for example failure of the thighbones in the legs to develop properly.

As previously mentioned there also, unfortunately, remain the risks of miscarriage (loss of pregnancy before 23 weeks) and stillbirth (the death of baby around the time of birth).

Problems for mum associated with GDM include high blood pressure and pre-eclampsia (along with the subsequent increased need for a caesarean section), and a subsequently increased risk of developing type 2 diabetes later in life – the conversion rate is around 3 per cent per year.

You must remember though that the vast majority of women with GDM go on to have a normal pregnancy with a healthy baby at the end of it. Modern antenatal care aims to reduce your risk of complications developing in the first place; hence all the monitoring, check-ups and gentle nagging.

8

Getting ready to deliver

After what had felt like an extremely long pregnancy, Elizabeth was more than ready for her baby to arrive.

The nursery was prepared, they had all the equipment, the car seat and the cot, and the bag was packed and by the front door. Elizabeth was anxious about giving birth and had spent a lot of time talking to friends about their own experiences and looking online at other people's descriptions of their good and bad birth stories.

She had spoken to Hannah, her midwife, who explained that they normally arranged for women with GDM who were on treatment to have their babies slightly earlier than the full 9 months (or 40 weeks) to limit the chances of complications occurring. Elizabeth was very keen to let the pregnancy go on for as long as possible and give her child the best chance of growing. She was worried that if the baby came out too soon there might be problems. Hannah the midwife, Ms Thallon the obstetrician, and Elizabeth discussed the timing of having an induction and they were able to agree on the best time. A date was set in the labour ward diary.

Elizabeth was initially upset that she wouldn't end up having a spontaneous delivery but understood that with GDM the antenatal team were in her corner and wanted the very best for her. Her birth plan included the option of a water birth, an epidural if necessary and for both her mum and Jon to be there. Julia, the diabetes nurse, told her about monitoring her blood sugars during labour and the possibility of having insulin through a drip if needed.

After all this time, everything was set.

How can I get ready for actually having my baby?

Preparing to give birth can be a stress-filled time for any woman. When GDM is added there are extra challenges to contend with. The following are important considerations for you and your team:

- Timing – when would be the safest stage of pregnancy?

- The actual mode of delivery – how is baby going to come out? By natural means, by being induced or by caesarean section?
- How do I make baby's delivery as natural as possible?
- What kind of painkillers can I have in labour?
- What is the best way of ensuring stable blood sugar levels throughout labour and delivery?

It is important that you discuss what will happen around the time of delivery well in advance with your antenatal team and your partner or friend or significant other, so that you are well prepared. A classic birth plan will include choices about different types of pain relief, advice on breastfeeding, a description of possible problems with the newborn baby and what the midwife will be doing straight after birth. Plus a discussion of the importance of good glycaemic control during labour and how to adjust your medication (if any) during this time. Some centres ask women fairly early on to think about a birthing wish list, but remember it may not be possible to follow all of this depending on the circumstances.

It is, however, very important to remember that you are the leader of your healthcare team!

Why have I been advised to have my baby in hospital rather than at home or in a midwife-led unit?

You will generally be advised to have your baby in hospital because of the risks associated with diabetes in pregnancy; it is best to deliver in a hospital that has the right facilities and back-up to look after sick babies and to support you 24 hours a day. This does not completely rule out giving birth elsewhere but it's important to have a discussion with your midwife about the potential risks and the delays in getting help if needed at a critical time. This is especially important if you are predicted to be having a large baby. Organizations such as the NCT are very keen to promote natural births and sometimes there can be guilt around not being able to have a completely natural, non-interventionist birth, so it's important to be realistic and talk with the specialists about the timing and place of birth. In addition, if you have previously had a caesarean section, you may still be okay to have a vaginal birth this time round. One does not always stop the other.

It may be that your birth experience is not the same as the one you'd hoped for. This can be difficult. Labour and birth often don't go to plan irrespective of GDM. Knowing what might happen can help you feel prepared.

Can I have a water birth?

Delivering in water can be a very positive experience and it is a good form of pain relief. Several centres do offer water births for women who have diabetes in pregnancy but often it depends on the availability of equipment and the need to monitor you regularly during labour. One key piece of kit is the **CTG** monitor (**cardio-tocograph**) which monitors the baby's heartbeat and the contractions of your uterus during pregnancy (it's also known as an electronic foetal monitor). This is strapped around your waist and helps the midwife to see if baby is okay during labour. However, not all centres have one that is waterproof – or it may be being used by somebody else! Therefore, on the day of delivery it may turn out that the water bath is not available or this lack of equipment prevents you from being able to have a water birth. Best to find out well in advance whether your obstetric unit provides this.

When will the baby need to be delivered?

Timing of delivery is an important issue. It was traditionally recognized that if the pregnancy of a woman with diabetes went on too long there would be an increased risk of complications such as obstructed labour (baby getting stuck) and stillbirth (the latter being related to degradation of the placenta). Therefore, the tendency has generally been to get baby out sooner to avoid the risk of these bad outcomes.

Your team will talk to you about tailoring the best plan for delivery at the appropriate time. It now seems the case in most places that if you have stable GDM, with no complications and being well-controlled on dietary intervention alone, then it's okay to let you go to full term (40 weeks). It would be very unlikely to let you go all the way to 41 weeks though.

If, however, you have been having problems with the diabetes control and are on medication or insulin injections, then there is a tendency to encourage earlier delivery and to get baby out via an induction of labour or caesarean section (depending on the circumstances and your preferences) around 37 to 38 weeks. If there are other problems such as high blood pressure or pre-eclampsia or evidence of growth restriction, then delivery may be planned even earlier.

What if labour starts by itself before 37 weeks?

If you have a spontaneous early labour, you might be offered treatment to delay the birth. Additionally, if baby comes early you should be given steroids, as mentioned in Chapter 7, in order to help the baby's lungs develop. The same rules will apply about the effects of steroids on blood glucose and it may be that if you are taking insulin, the dose will need to be increased and the sugar levels monitored more closely.

How will baby be monitored during birth?

The piece of kit used to monitor baby (the CTG or cardio-tocograph, described earlier in this chapter) consists of two sensors which are strapped to your bump by a piece of elastic or material. This continuously keeps a record of baby's heart rate during labour and can also pick up when the uterus is undergoing a contraction. This can help with guiding you when to push and makes sure that the baby is not becoming distressed.

What do you mean by induction of labour?

This describes the artificial triggering of labour. This is not an uncommon process and is done in one in five pregnancies in the UK. It is usually done if baby is overdue or there is some sort of risk to baby's health. Before labour is induced you might be offered a membrane or cervical sweep in order to bring on labour. This involves the midwife or obstetrician sweeping a finger around the bottom of the cervix during an internal vaginal examination. It helps to separate the membranes between the fluid sac surrounding baby and your cervix and this can stimulate the hormones which bring on labour.

If this is unsuccessful, induction of labour will take place in the maternity unit, involving the insertion of a special tablet (pessary) or gel (containing prostaglandins) into the vagina in order to bring on the contractions of labour. It helps to accelerate the normal labour process but can sometimes take up to 24 hours to get to work.

If it's unsuccessful, then you may be offered an amniotomy. This method of labour induction involves the artificial breaking of the waters during an internal examination (sometimes using a small hook). This then stimulates the beginning of labour.

Alternatively, if you are still not in labour then an IV (intravenous) drip can be set up to deliver hormones (called Syntocinon) into your system to bring about labour. Once labour starts it should go ahead normally, but it can sometimes take a while to get going.

Induced labour, however, may be more painful due to the force of the contractions and women may be more likely to need a spinal or epidural anaesthetic.

What happens with a caesarean section?

A caesarean is an operation to get baby out. It may be used in circumstances when it is likely to be difficult to deliver normally, such as with a very large baby: if the placenta is in the way of the birth canal, if baby is upside down (breech) or if the mother has had two or more previous caesarean sections (in this situation there is a risk of the previous operation scars coming apart).

It involves making a cut in the lower part of your tummy and then the uterus and is usually done under a local anaesthetic where the lower part of your body is numbed. The operation takes around 40 to 50 minutes. The obstetrician will explain the procedure to you and ask you to give formal consent, after explaining the risks versus the benefits. An anaesthetist will give you a regional anaesthetic to numb the lower part of your body.

The complications of a caesarean include bleeding and infection and it takes longer to recover from than a vaginal birth. The muscles in the lower abdominal wall and the scarring need to heal up. You may well have a catheter put into your bladder to help you wee and you'll also be given regular painkillers – don't be afraid to ask for more! You may end up staying in hospital for 3 to 4 days after delivery and will be unable to drive a car for a few weeks as well.

What happens when the baby is being delivered?

Now you're at the final hurdle, it's annoying to find out that your blood glucose levels will be checked even more frequently. During established labour it's generally the case that your blood glucose level will be checked every 30 to 60 minutes to make sure that it stays at a safe level – generally thought to be below 7.0 mmol/l.

The rationale behind this is to prevent neonatal hypoglycaemia. If baby goes from a high glucose environment inside mum and pops out into the outside world where the baby no longer has access to mum's glucose, then the baby can suddenly suffer a hypo (baby will be making plenty of insulin of his or her own to deal with mum's high glucose coming through the umbilical cord) and become unwell. Baby may even need to be taken off to the special care unit to be treated with glucose.

If your glucose level is persistently greater than 7.0 then the normal management is to start you on an IV drip with insulin going into you directly in order to control the sugar levels.

Will my baby be checked for diabetes when he or she is born?

The baby will have a special blood test for its glucose levels soon after birth (usually within the first 4 hours) to make sure that they have not gone too low. You will be advised to start feeding your baby as soon as possible after delivery (within the first half an hour) and then every couple of hours after that to help your baby's glucose level stay in the safe range.

What if my baby has a hypo?

If the baby's blood glucose is persistently on the low side, it may need to be fed through a special feeding tube or given a drip to help bring the glucose level up to normal. This can happen as baby's own insulin levels may still be on the high side in order to combat the high sugar levels coming from mum. Rarely, severe hypoglycaemia can cause the baby to have a fit. Prompt feeding and/or IV glucose solution can bring the baby's glucose levels back into the normal range. Sometimes baby may need to temporarily go to the special care baby unit to make sure that he or she is well.

Will I continue to have gestational diabetes once the baby is out?

Women who have had GDM should stay in hospital for the first 24 hours following delivery to check that the baby is feeding well and that its glucose levels remain good.

Once your baby has been delivered and the placenta has come out, then your metabolism goes back to normal. You are no longer doing the hard work of growing a human and the GDM will simply disappear in the vast majority of women.

Do I need to continue with my medication?

After the birth you can stop taking all the tablets or insulin injections for your diabetes. If you have been taking a long acting insulin, it maybe that you are advised not to take this the night before delivery (or to take a reduced dose) in order to stop you from becoming hypoglycaemic when you are no longer diabetic!

Do I need to carry on measuring my blood sugar levels?

Your blood glucose levels will be checked to make sure that they are back to normal (the non-pregnancy target range is less strict) a few times over the next 24–48 hours following delivery to make sure that everything has stabilized.

Will GDM stop me from breastfeeding?

No. There should be no problems. Remember to keep up your food intake however, as breastfeeding is a demanding business.

What happens if the diabetes doesn't go away after the birth?

Don't panic. Diabetes in the non-pregnant state is a different kettle of fish. Depending on your situation and the state of your blood sugars it may be that you can be managed with diet and lifestyle alone rather than medication, if it's thought that you have type 2 diabetes. Some patients do turn out to have undiagnosed type 1 diabetes and remain dependent on insulin following the birth of their baby. If the diabetes persists then the team will make sure that you get all of the right treatment, information and follow-up.

Will I need to have another glucose tolerance test after the baby is born?

We need to make sure that the diabetes has gone away completely once baby has been delivered. Diabetologists still continue to argue about the best way to actually diagnose diabetes!

The latest NICE guidance recommends that a fasting blood glucose test takes place at some point between 6 and 12 weeks after birth. A fasting blood test (drawn from a vein) rather than a finger prick test is a more accurate way of assessing your baseline blood sugar level and will show whether you are normal, have glucose intolerance (pre-diabetes), or continue to have high blood glucose levels and full-blown diabetes.

Normally you will not be offered another oral glucose tolerance test although some centres do do this to confirm the situation, or alternatively use the HbA1c blood test.

Make sure you don't miss the follow-up test. Coping with a new baby can be an exhausting business, but it's important to confirm that the diabetes has gone away and that mum remains well.

9

After the birth

Elizabeth felt a huge wave of relief. Baby was out, a beautiful little girl called Robin, weighing in at 8 pounds 2 ounces. Labour had been long and uncomfortable but there had been no complications and everything had gone to plan.

During labour she did end up on a drip but knew to expect this. And when Robin's blood sugar was checked after her first feed her glucose level was normal, she seemed happy and dribbly and fell fast asleep on top of Elizabeth.

Jon brought a surprise for Elizabeth, something she had been craving for several months – chocolate digestives. She ate almost the whole packet and enjoyed every mouthful. The GDM was now gone and she was back to normal – until the next time.

Will I be checked again in future for diabetes?

Yes. GDM is a noted risk factor for type 2 diabetes. The current standard of care is to make sure that all women who have had GDM receive a blood test for HbA1c or fasting blood glucose 6 to 12 weeks after delivering their baby and then every year in order to screen them for the disease. Figure 9.1 shows how your doctor will interpret your HbA1c or fasting blood glucose results.

What are the other types of diabetes?

Type 1 diabetes   This is caused by an immune system attack on the pancreas which causes almost complete destruction of the insulin-producing cells. This diagnosis should be apparent during pregnancy but it may not be until after delivery that it is properly identified – baby is out but the blood sugars go very high without the insulin. If type 1 diabetes is confirmed then insulin treatment may need to continue for life, as without it you can become very unwell.

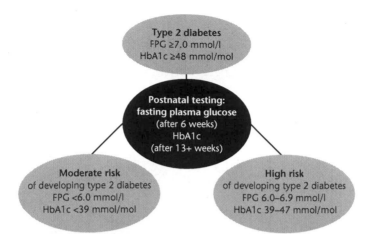

Figure 9.1 Interpretation of postnatal testing following GDM
FPG: fasting plasma glucose
Note Reproduced with permission from the *British Journal of Diabetes*

Type 2 diabetes This is the most common form of diabetes and relates to insulin resistance. It is caused by many factors including genetics, ethnicity, BMI and lifestyle.

Polycystic ovarian syndrome (PCOS) This is commonly associated with type 2 diabetes as the underlying mechanism of insulin resistance is similar. PCOS is made worse by being overweight and is associated with erratic periods, excess annoying hair growth and an imbalance in the levels of oestrogen and testosterone.

Steroid-induced diabetes Certain medications such as steroids can interfere with how the body handles carbohydrates. If you notice that blood sugars are high or there are symptoms of diabetes, it may be that prednisolone or some other form of steroid (including inhalers) could be making this worse.

Secondary diabetes This can occur if there is some form of direct damage to the pancreas such as trauma or an operation, pancreatitis (inflammation of the pancreas due to a variety of causes including alcohol excess) or cystic fibrosis.

Monogenic diabetes Sometimes called maturity onset diabetes of the young or MODY, this occurs when a single gene mutation is passed on which can cause unusual forms of diabetes. Sometimes it can present like type 2 diabetes or be mistaken for type 1 diabetes. One of the key factors is its tendency to run in families. If there are two or more first degree relatives (parents or siblings) who develop diabetes at an early age (under 35 years old) then there could be a genetic cause. Things to look out for are persistently elevated fasting blood glucose levels (but normal after eating), kidney problems such as cysts, or neurological features, and if these are present then it is worth considering the diagnosis.

What happens when I am planning future pregnancies?

The team looking after you will make sure that you get screened for diabetes in future and if you become pregnant you'll receive testing for GDM from an early stage. If it is negative in the early stages of pregnancy you will then have a repeat test every month during the pregnancy until it becomes positive (or not).

In the meantime, you will be given advice about your lifestyle factors, such as helping to make your diet better, maintaining a healthy weight and taking regular, effective exercise. If you are actively trying to get pregnant then 5 milligrams of folic acid per day is recommended.

How do I reduce my future risk of developing gestational diabetes?

You can reduce your future risk of developing GDM by doing all of the common-sense stuff, which is easy to describe but more difficult to put into practice once you are the parent of a young child. It can be tricky to find the time to look after yourself. Consider GDM a warning shot for later life as some simple changes could help to avoid a lifetime of problems.

- Being physically active 30 minutes a day for 5 days a week, e.g. yoga, jogging, swimming and walking regularly.
- Eating healthily – making good food choices and eating smaller

portions which are high in fibre and low in sugar and fat (by now hopefully you are used to looking at food labels). This includes eating five portions of fruit and vegetables per day.

- Stopping smoking.
- Avoiding weight gain in pregnancy and losing weight after pregnancy if you are overweight. Find out what your BMI is and set yourself a target weight.

Of those women with a history of GDM who reach their ideal body weight after delivery, fewer than 1 in 4 eventually go on to develop type 2 diabetes.

Will my baby get diabetes?

Even though you had GDM in pregnancy, this will not cause diabetes in your baby. However, your child is at higher risk for developing type 2 diabetes later in life. As baby grows up, sensible things like having a healthy family diet, keeping a healthy weight and getting regular physical activity can help to reduce that risk.

If baby was on the large side at birth, then he or she is at a higher risk of childhood and adult obesity (being very overweight). Big babies are also at greater risk of getting type 2 diabetes and often get it at an earlier age (younger than 30).

What else should I do after delivery?

There are some specific concerns for the early care of women with GDM following delivery. You don't have to worry too much if you are struggling to breastfeed your baby, but exclusive breastfeeding for your baby does have profound short-term and long-term health benefits for infants. A form of contraception should be chosen that does not increase your risk of glucose intolerance. If the diabetes does persist after delivery then you'll be given information about the non-pregnancy glucose targets and have your blood pressure, urine protein and cholesterol checked.

Useful addresses

There are several good sources of support and information to help you.

BabyCentre
Website: www.babycentre.co.uk

See <www.babycentre.co.uk/a2058/gestational-diabetes>.

Diabetes UK
Macleod House
10 Parkway
London NW1 7AA
Tel.: 0345 123 2399
Fax: 020 7424 1001
Website: https://www.diabetes.org.uk

See <https://www.diabetes.org.uk/Guide-to-diabetes/What-is-diabetes/
Gestational-diabetes/>.

Mumsnet
Studio 6
Deane House Studios
Greenwood Place
Highgate Road
London NW5 1LB
Website: www.mumsnet.com

See <www.mumsnet.com/pregnancy/gestational-diabetes>.

Royal College of Obstetricians and Gynaecologists
27 Sussex Place
Regent's Park
London NW1 4RG
Tel.: 020 7772 6200
Fax: 020 7723 0575
Website: https://www.rcog.org.uk

See <https://www.rcog.org.uk/en/patients/patient-leaflets/
gestational-diabetes/>.

Notes

The new NICE guidance NG3

Previously the diagnosis and management of GDM have been plagued by different definitions and management plans. We are still learning the best approach to treating people with diabetes in pregnancy. There remain several unknowns, so most treatment advice is based on best practice guidelines, common sense and a commitment to safety.

In February 2015, the updated NICE guidelines were published on the management of diabetes in pregnancy. The diagnostic criteria for making the diagnosis and the treatment targets were adjusted to what is included in this book, along with a whole raft of other useful advice. More flexibility is now offered around the timing of delivery based on individual circumstances, for example.

The seminal Australian Carbohydrate Intolerance Study in Pregnant Women suggested a reduction in serious perinatal complications from 4 per cent to 1 per cent with treatment of GDM. This is a significant reduction and provides reassurance to clinicians in the antenatal ward that the work we do makes a difference.

Index